Talking Health

Talking Health

A New Way to Communicate about Public Health

Edited by

Mark R. Miller, Brian C. Castrucci, Rachel Locke,
Julia Haskins, and Grace A. Castillo

de Beaumont
BOLD SOLUTIONS FOR HEALTHIER COMMUNITIES.

OXFORD
UNIVERSITY PRESS

OXFORD
UNIVERSITY PRESS

Oxford University Press is a department of the University of Oxford. It furthers the University's objective of excellence in research, scholarship, and education by publishing worldwide. Oxford is a registered trade mark of Oxford University Press in the UK and certain other countries.

Published in the United States of America by Oxford University Press
198 Madison Avenue, New York, NY 10016, United States of America.

Library of Congress Cataloging-in-Publication Data
Names: Miller, Mark (Mark Richard), editor. | Castrucci, Brian C., editor. |
Locke, Rachel, editor. | Haskins, Julia, editor. | Castillo, Grace A., editor. |
de Beaumont Foundation, issuing body.
Title: Talking health : a new way to communicate about public health /
edited by Mark R. Miller, Brian C. Castrucci, Rachel Locke,
Julia Haskins, and Grace A. Castillo.
Other titles: Talking health (Miller) | Reframing public health
communication to win hearts and minds
Description: New York, NY : Oxford University Press ; [Bethesda, Maryland]:
de Beaumont Foundation, [2022] | Includes bibliographical
references and index.
Identifiers: LCCN 2022005957 (print) | LCCN 2022005958 (ebook) |
ISBN 9780197528464 (paperback) | ISBN 9780197528488 (epub) |
ISBN 9780197528495
Subjects: MESH: Public Health Administration—methods | Communication |
Community-Institutional Relations | Intersectoral Collaboration
Classification: LCC RA418 (print) | LCC RA418 (ebook) | NLM WA 525 |
DDC 362.1—dc23/eng/20220404
LC record available at https://lccn.loc.gov/2022005957
LC ebook record available at https://lccn.loc.gov/2022005958

DOI: 10.1093/oso/9780197528464.001.0001

Printed by Marquis, Canada

Contents

Part III. Bringing Public Health to Life

Acknowledgments

The editors would like to acknowledge and thank the many people who contributed to this book and the initiative that inspired it, Public Health Reaching Across Sectors (PHRASES). First, we'd like to thank each of the authors who took the time to share their expertise and perspectives. We were fortunate to be able to include such prominent leaders in health and communication, and we know readers will benefit from their insights based on their personal experiences.

The de Beaumont Foundation and the Aspen Institute's Health, Medicine & Society Program launched the PHRASES initiative in 2017, and its tools and resources were released in July 2020. Intended to help public health professionals communicate more effectively about public health and form stronger partnerships, PHRASES would not have been possible without advice and guidance of a dream team of experts. An advisory board was chaired by Karen DeSalvo, MD, MPH, MSc, and Soledad O'Brien, and its members included John Auerbach, MBA; Raymond J. Baxter, PhD; Richard Berke; Gary M. Cohen, MBA; John Dreyzehner, MD, MPH, FACOEM; Sandro Galea,

MD, DrPH; Jackie Judd; and Joe Reardon, JD. They generously shared their firsthand experience and knowledge, providing us with lessons learned and a vision for improving public health communication.

The work of the FrameWorks Institute and Hattaway Communications forms the backbone of this book. FrameWorks conducted a detailed audit and interviewed leaders in business, health care, education, and housing to evaluate perceptions of the public health field. They then developed the framing, metaphors, and many of the tools that are featured in this book. Hattaway Communications built on the FrameWorks research to develop and test messaging with a broader audience, and their practical guides for communication are incorporated into several chapters. We are grateful to Nat Kendall-Taylor and his team at the FrameWorks Institute and Doug Hattaway and his team at Hattaway Communications.

In addition to the editors, many other de Beaumont Foundation employees contributed to PHRASES and this book in a number of ways, and we are grateful for their support. We also want to thank Ruth J. Katz, executive director of the Aspen Institute's Health, Medicine & Society Program, and the many Aspen employees and contractors who helped lead the PHRASES initiative and helped form the vision for this book.

Finally, this book would not have been possible without the support of Dr. James B. Sprague, chairman of the de Beaumont Foundation Board of Directors, and our founder, the late Pete de Beaumont.

About the Editors

Mark R. Miller, Vice President of Communications at the de Beaumont Foundation, leads strategic communications to support the foundation's mission, initiatives, and partners, applying his experience in philanthropy, journalism, health care, and government to improve the health of communities and people. In 2018, he won the ACE Award from PR Daily and Ragan Communications as the year's top nonprofit communications professional. Throughout his career, Mark has advanced political, nonprofit, and corporate missions in leadership positions at the Case Foundation, the White House, Children's National Hospital, the National Governors Association, and AmeriCorps. He was also a senior vice president at Powell Tate, the Washington office of global PR agency Weber Shandwick. He combines traditional communications skills with an expertise in digital strategies to create solutions that deliver measurable results and spark social change. His writing has appeared in numerous blogs, websites, and publications, and for several years he was the reggae reporter for *The Washington Post*. He earned his BA in English and journalism from James Madison University.

Brian C. Castrucci, DrPH, is an epidemiologist, public health practitioner, and president and chief executive officer of the de Beaumont Foundation. Prior to joining de Beaumont, Brian worked for a decade as an applied epidemiologist and held leadership positions in several state and local governmental public health agencies. Applying what he learned in his public health practice, Brian has led the foundation to the forefront of issues such as integrating primary care and public health, assessing the governmental public health workforce, and prioritizing partnerships and policies to solve the nation's most complex health challenges. He is a sought-after resource on public health issues across television, radio, and print media and is an accomplished public health researcher with nearly ninety peer-reviewed scientific publications that have garnered more than 2,700 citations. He has also co-edited five books and written chapters for several others. Brian earned his doctorate in Public Health Leadership from the Gillings School of Global Public Health at the University of North Carolina at Chapel Hill and a Master of Arts degree in Sociomedical Sciences from Columbia University. He earned a Bachelor of Arts in political science with the greatest distinction from North Carolina State University.

Rachel Locke, MPH, as a senior program associate at the de Beaumont Foundation, was responsible for assessing the impact of the foundation's programs and managing grants across the foundation's portfolio. She led programs and projects that focused on public health communications, building local and state governmental public health workforce capacity and advancing public health policy. Previously she held positions at the Cancer Free Economy Network and the Big Cities Health Coalition and completed the Association of Schools and Programs of Public Health (ASPPH) Philanthropy Fellowship at the foundation. Rachel received her MPH in Environmental Health from the Columbia University Mailman School of Public Health, where she completed her Certificate in Toxicology.

Julia Haskins is a communications associate at the de Beaumont Foundation, where she develops and implements a wide range of editorial strategies to extend the foundation's reach, influence, and impact. Julia previously was a staff writer at the Association of American Medical Colleges, where she wrote about trends and research in academic medicine for the association's digital news publication, *AAMCNews*. She also worked as a reporter for *The Nation's Health*, the official newspaper of the American Public Health Association, covering public health and member news. She holds a Bachelor of Science in journalism from the Medill School of Journalism, Media, Integrated Marketing Communications at Northwestern University.

Grace A. Castillo, MPH, is a public health practitioner and health writer. She is particularly interested in public health infrastructure, science communication, and non-communicable diseases. As a program associate at the de Beaumont Foundation, she focused on project management for book publications. She has also volunteered with the Virginia Medical Reserve Corps. Previously, she worked for the Equity Research and Innovation Center (ERIC) as a student research intern. Grace graduated from the Yale School of Public Health's Chronic Disease Epidemiology Department with a Certificate in Regulatory Affairs. While completing her Master of Public Health, Grace interned with the Patient-Centered Outcomes Research Institute, where she worked with the Research Infrastructure team. Grace earned her BA in English from Yale University.

Contributors

Rose Arce is executive producer of Soledad O'Brien Productions. She spent fifteen years as a senior producer and documentary filmmaker at CNN, for whom she produced eight feature-length documentaries and won an Emmy. She began her TV career at CBS News and WCBS, where she won two Emmys for spot news and investigative reporting. She was previously a print reporter at the *NY Daily News* and *NY Newsday*, where she shared a Pulitzer Prize with her colleagues.

Maureen Byrnes, MPA, is a member of the faculty in the Milken Institute School of Public Health at The George Washington University. She has served in leadership positions in the federal government, philanthropy, and the nonprofit sector, including as director of the Health and Human Services program at The Pew Charitable Trusts and as the executive director of Human Rights First. Maureen worked with Senator Lowell Weicker as the staff director of the U.S. Senate Appropriations Subcommittee on Labor, HHS, Education and Related Agencies to provide early government funding to address the HIV epidemic. Later she served as executive director of the National Commission on AIDS, the first congressionally mandated independent commission to address the challenges associated with the HIV epidemic.

Karen DeSalvo, MD, MPH, MSc, is chief health officer at Google, where she leads a team of health professionals who provide guidance for the development of health research, products, and services across Google. Karen's career has focused on improving health and eliminating disparities, and she leans on deep experience working at the intersection of medicine, public health, and information technology. Before joining Google, she was National Coordinator for Health Information Technology and Assistant Secretary for Health (Acting) in the Obama Administration. During her time at the U.S. Department of Health and Human Services, Karen focused on creating a more consumer-oriented, transparent, and value-based health system. She also served as the New Orleans Health Commissioner following Hurricane Katrina. She was previously Vice Dean for Community Affairs and Health Policy at the Tulane School of Medicine, where she was a practicing internal medicine physician, educator, researcher, and leader. She serves on the Council of the National Academy of Medicine.

Anna Duin, a former content marketing specialist at mySidewalk, is a marketer, writer, and mother. She believes that action begins with data, and that by knowing your audience better than anyone else, you can speak to their pain, position your brand as their guide, and be the thought leader they need. Her expertise is in inbound and content marketing. Simply put, she creates content to drive measurable business results. Anna attended the University of Missouri-Kansas City, where she studied psychology. She loves finding new ways to solve problems, making a difference, and chasing after her two boys.

Doug Hattaway, president of Hattaway Communications, helps visionary leaders and organizations use the power of strategy, science, and storytelling to achieve ambitious goals for people and the planet. He pioneered an approach known as Aspirational Communication, which was featured in a *Stanford Social Innovation Review* cover story about the historic marriage equality movement and Truth anti-smoking campaign, which "transformed public attitudes by connecting their causes to the personal aspirations of their audiences." Doug has three decades of experience working with leaders at the highest levels of U.S. politics and government, international organizations and NGOs, cutting-edge businesses, and the world's largest foundations.

Ruth J. Katz, JD, MPH, is vice president and executive director of the Health, Medicine & Society (HMS) Program at the Aspen Institute, an education and policy studies organization based in Washington, DC. HMS signature initiatives include the Aspen Health Strategy

Group, the Sabin-Aspen Vaccine Science & Policy Group, and Aspen Ideas Health. Ruth joined the Aspen Institute after serving from 2009 to 2013 as chief public health counsel (Democratic staff) with the Committee on Energy and Commerce in the U.S. House of Representatives, which has legislative jurisdiction over domestic health programs, including Medicare, Medicaid, the National Institutes of Health, the Centers for Disease Control and Prevention, the Food and Drug Administration, and national health reform efforts. Prior to her work with the committee, Ruth was the Walter G. Ross Professor of Health Policy at the Milken Institute School of Public Health at The George Washington University and served as the dean from 2003 to 2008. From 1997 to 2003, she was associate dean for administration at the Yale University School of Medicine, where she also held appointments in the departments of Internal Medicine (General Medicine) and Epidemiology and Public Health as an assistant professor. A magna cum laude graduate of the University of Pennsylvania, Ruth holds a law degree from Emory University and a Master of Public Health from Harvard University.

Nat Kendall-Taylor, PhD, is chief executive officer at the FrameWorks Institute, a research think tank in Washington, DC. He leads a multidisciplinary team in conducting research on public understanding and framing of social issues and supporting nonprofit organizations to implement findings. A psychological anthropologist, Nat publishes widely on communications research in the popular and professional press and lectures frequently in the United States and abroad. He is a senior fellow at the Center on the Developing Child at Harvard University, a visiting professor at the Child Study Center at Yale School of Medicine, and a fellow at the British-American Project.

Sarah Martin, PhD, is vice president of Health Solutions at mySidewalk, a technology firm specializing in data storytelling for community change. She was previously the deputy director of the Kansas City, Missouri Health Department and an assistant professor of health services research at the Bloch School of Management at the University of Missouri, Kansas City. Sarah received a Master of Public Policy, a Master of Public Health, and a PhD in public policy from the University of California, Berkeley.

Soledad O'Brien is an award-winning documentarian, journalist, speaker, author, and philanthropist and the founder of Soledad O'Brien Productions, a multi-platform media production company dedicated to uncovering and producing empowering untold stories that look at the often divisive issues of race, class, wealth, opportunity, and poverty. She anchors and produces the Hearst TV political magazine program "Matter of Fact with Soledad O'Brien," which reaches 95% of U.S. households and has more than a million viewers weekly. She also hosts the Quake Media podcast "Very Opinionated with Soledad O'Brien" and is a correspondent for HBO's "Real Sports with Bryant Gumbel." Soledad O'Brien Productions recently produced the series "Disrupt and Dismantle" for BET, "Who Killed My Son?" for Discovery+, and the much-lauded documentaries "Hungry to Learn" and "Outbreak: The First Response." As a thought leader, Soledad has over 1.3 million Twitter followers and is a frequent op-ed contributor to news outlets including the *New York Times* and *Huffington Post.* Throughout her storied career, she has anchored news shows on CNN, MSNBC, and NBC, and reported for Fox, A&E, Oxygen, Nat Geo, PBS NewsHour, WebMD, and Al Jazeera America, among others. Her work has been recognized with three Emmy awards, two George Foster Peabody Awards, three Gracie Awards, two Cine Awards, and an Alfred I. DuPont Award.

Moriah Robins, MPH, is a senior research associate at the de Beaumont Foundation. Her focus is on the Public Health Workforce Interests and Needs Survey (PH WINS), the only nationally representative survey of the state and local government workforce. Previously, Moriah served as a research associate on the PHRASES project (Public Health Reaching Across Sectors), a partnership between the de Beaumont Foundation and the Aspen Institute. There she designed and managed the PHRASES Fellows, a program aimed at training public health professionals in framing and communicating the value of public health in a way that resonates with decision-makers in other sectors. She earned her MPH in Global Health Program Design, Monitoring, and Evaluation from the Milken Institute School of Public Health at The George Washington University. Moriah holds a BS in chemistry from the University of Maryland in College Park, Maryland.

Eric Zimmermann, vice president at Quadrant Strategies and former director at Hattaway Communications, is a communications strategist who uses audience research to help organizations change the narrative on complex issues. He has spent more than a decade helping clients in government, politics, business, and philanthropy develop research-based brand, message, and public affairs strategies. He has particular interest in using insights from cognitive science, psychology, and other fields to understand audience motivations and craft effective messages. Prior to joining Quadrant, he served as director of strategy at Hattaway Communications, where he led national and international research, narrative development, and communications training programs for advocacy coalitions, global philanthropies, and mission-driven businesses. He has a deep background in both public health and health care, having worked extensively on vaccine confidence, infectious diseases, and the social determinants of health. Previously, Eric worked at Benenson Strategy Group, where he managed quantitative and qualitative research for House and Senate campaigns, advocacy organizations, and Fortune 500 companies. He began his career as a staff writer for *The Hill* newspaper, where he covered Congress and campaigns. Eric graduated from Stanford University with a bachelor's degree in history.

Introduction: Good Health Depends on Better Communication and Stronger Partnerships

RUTH J. KATZ, MAUREEN BYRNES, AND BRIAN C. CASTRUCCI

PUBLIC HEALTH POLICIES AND PRACTICES HAVE an impact on most everyone's daily life. Practitioners monitor emerging infections and rates of chronic disease, conduct food safety and restaurant inspections, and work to reduce the likelihood of injuries, among dozens of other complex, science-based responsibilities designed to improve the public's health and well-being.

From 1900 to 1999, life expectancy in the United States increased by 30 years, and according to the Centers for Disease Control and Prevention (CDC), public health interventions account for 25 of those years.[1,2] However, few people—even public health professionals—can describe public health

Ruth J. Katz, Maureen Byrnes, and Brian C. Castrucci, *Introduction* In: *Talking Health*. Edited by:
Mark R. Miller, Brian C. Castrucci, Rachel Locke, Julia Haskins, and Grace A. Castillo, Oxford University Press.
© de Beaumont Foundation 2022. DOI: 10.1093/oso/9780197528464.003.0001

in a meaningful and consistent way that is easy to understand. Forming effective partnerships and creating healthier communities must start with clear and consistent communication about what public health is and why it matters.

The COVID-19 pandemic has powerfully revealed the indispensable role that public health plays in protecting the nation's health, security, and economic strength. For decades before the pandemic, state and local health departments experienced repeated declines in funding and staffing.[3] Despite this underinvestment in prevention and preparation, public health leaders formed the core of the nation's response to the pandemic. Working with the federal government, leaders in state and local governmental public health agencies made critical decisions that impacted businesses, schools, faith communities, and nearly every other aspect of our lives.

However, from the earliest days of the pandemic, the response was framed as a false dichotomy between saving lives and saving livelihoods, which fed directly into the country's existing political polarization. Public health practitioners were often cast as anti-freedom and anti-economy government agents, and threats and harassment contributed, in part, to the resignation of hundreds of public health leaders and staff.[4-5] Misinformation and polarization colluded to limit the effectiveness of public health messaging and science-based interventions. Adding to this was the reality that with a novel virus, recommendations could change on a weekly or even daily basis, depending on data such as infection rates and new information about viral transmission. Where there was success—acceptance and compliance with public health guidance about social distancing, mask-wearing, vaccination, travel, and other issues—it was dependent on the credibility of state and local public health leaders and the strength of the relationships they had built in their communities prior to the pandemic. Unfortunately, when these leaders needed to recommend temporarily closing businesses and schools and suspending religious, sporting, and entertainment gatherings, they often lacked the partnerships needed to engender familiarity and trust from those most impacted by these actions.

This book was not written in response to the COVID-19 pandemic or the public health challenges it exposed. The work that led to the creation of this book began in 2017 as a collaboration between the de Beaumont Foundation and the Aspen Institute's Health, Medicine & Society Program to help public health professionals create the vibrant, structured, cross-sector partnerships needed to support healthy, thriving communities. While the development of the tools, metaphors, and messaging included in this book began long before anyone had heard of COVID-19, these resources were needed before the pandemic, and they are even more critical now.

Communication skills have been a consistent challenge for public health practitioners. In 2015, Katherine Lyon Daniel, then the associate director of communication at the CDC, suggested that "public health" may be a "dirty word" to people not in the field.[6,7] She referenced a CDC Foundation study that found the term "public health" tested poorly among non–public health professionals.[6,7] "If we keep talking to people in the same words that we want to use," she said, "then we're not going to be understood. . . . We have to adapt."[6,7]

In the 2017 Public Health Workforce Interests and Needs Survey, conducted by the de Beaumont Foundation and the Association of State and Territorial Health Officials, state and local health department staff identified communication as one of the most important skills in their daily work.[8] More important, nearly one-fifth of respondents reported that they needed to improve their communication skills.[9]

After identifying communication as an important need in public health, the de Beaumont Foundation and the Aspen Institute's Health, Medicine & Society Program created the Public Health Reaching Across Sectors initiative (PHRASES), which was designed to provide public health leaders with a toolkit for promoting their field as an essential partner in the work of many other sectors to improve community health. However, as the work began, we quickly learned that leaders in housing, health care, business, and education held a narrow and often negative perception of public health professionals as community leaders and strategists. In-depth interviews with sector leaders conducted by the Frameworks Institute, a non-profit think tank that helps change conversations about social issues, confirmed that leaders from these sectors did not appreciate the value that public health departments could add to strategic collaborations to strengthen communities. The sector leaders participating in the interviews thought of public health professionals as highly bureaucratic specialists who performed traditional roles of regulators, data crunchers, and health service providers. To them, public health professionals were "book smart," impractical researchers or siloed bureaucrats who were unsuited to address "real-world" challenges. The findings from this research are summarized in Chapter 6.

This book is intended for public health professionals and any others who communicate about public health. From officials at the CDC to frontline professionals in local health departments, most public health practitioners have not had formal training in communicating about public health. While they have been trained in medicine, policy, or some other discipline, most health professionals have never had to "sell" ideas to uninformed or skeptical partners. The insights, tools, and resources included in this book can provide a first step toward better communications and stronger partnerships.

This book highlights the value of strong communication and the critical importance of framing, messaging, and storytelling. It can help professionals avoid messages that backfire, answer challenging questions, reframe public health assumptions, and draw on the power of anecdotes while sharing important data. For those who want to develop their skills further, additional tools and trainings can be found at www.phrases.org, which is accessible at no cost.

In the aftermath of the COVID-19 pandemic, it is critical for public health professionals of all backgrounds to strengthen their communication skills. The next public health emergency—natural, climate related, or manufactured—is coming. All sectors and all populations stand to gain by capitalizing on the public health field's expertise and leadership. Now is the time to be bold and shatter the norms of what public health professionals are expected to do. *Talking Health* and PHRASES provide crucial resources for those who are ready change how public health is viewed and valued in our nation.

Part I
Why Public Health Needs to Do Better

1

Perceptions of Public Health: The Gaps Between Insiders and Other Leaders

MORIAH ROBINS

Introduction

The perceptions that other sectors have about public health often stand in the way of effective collaboration. Public health professionals have long understood the interconnectedness of health and other aspects of our communities and our lives. However, leaders in other sectors often are unaware of the ways their priorities are affected by health—or the ways that public health professionals can help them achieve their strategic goals. Since collaboration is a two-way street, this lack of a shared vision and understanding can impede the potential for strong community partnerships.

Building a common mission must start with an understanding of current perceptions and obstacles. That is why the de Beaumont Foundation and the Aspen Institute's Health,

Moriah Robins, *Perceptions of Public Health* In: *Talking Health.* Edited by: Mark R. Miller, Brian C. Castrucci, Rachel Locke, Julia Haskins, and Grace A. Castillo, Oxford University Press.

Medicine & Society Program, through the PHRASES initiative, partnered with the FrameWorks Institute to discover the gaps between public health experts and leaders in housing, education, business, and health systems. This chapter summarizes the findings of the "Map the Gaps" report that resulted from in-depth interviews with these community leaders. The full report is available at https://www.phrases.org/wp-content/uploads/2020/07/Aspen-PHRASES-MTG-Report-2019.pdf.

In order to identify the gaps in understanding about public health, FrameWorks first talked to experts in public health. Through sixteen one-on-one phone interviews with researchers, practitioners, and policy experts, FrameWorks asked questions such as the following:

- What should leaders in sectors outside of public health know about health?
- What should leaders in sectors outside of public health know about public health?
- What value does public health bring to other sectors?
- What would be helpful in forging partnerships between public health and other sectors?

FrameWorks then conducted thirty-eight in-person, in-depth interviews with leaders in the housing, education, business, and health systems sectors. That research focused on these questions:

- What is health?
- What is public health?

- What shapes health?
- How is health connected to the work of other sectors?
- How do cross-sector collaborations work?
- How do other sectors think about data?

In brief, the FrameWorks research showed that leaders in housing, education, business, and health systems associate the field of public health with a narrow set of traditional functions related to preventing disease and protecting health (Figure 1.1). They generally do not recognize the value of public health leaders as effective partners. Simply put, these sectors often see public health professionals as "book smart" but not as strategists. The research, however, did identify several areas of shared understanding and mission; those overlaps are discussed at the end of this chapter.

The views of leaders and professionals outside public health

Leaders from the sectors of housing, education, and health systems, as well as leaders and professionals from the business sector, draw on a complex set of professional cultural models to make sense of health, public health, and cross-sector collaborations. To identify these models, FrameWorks researchers analyzed transcripts from the thirty-eight interviews with sector leaders and two peer discourse sessions with business professionals.

The research revealed the following implicit understandings and assumptions, among others.

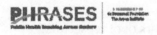

Gaps at a Glance

Key differences between how **experts in public health** and **leaders in other sectors** think about the topics of health, public health, and cross-sector collaboration.

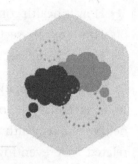

Mapping the Gaps between How Public Health Experts and Leaders in Other Sectors View Public Health and Cross-Sector Collaboration

Gaps in understanding	Experts in public health	Leaders in other sectors *(Housing, education, health systems, and business)*
Health, as a general concept is understood as...	A positive state of integrated well-being	The absence of illness
Social determinants of health refers to...	The protective factors and risk factors that promote or undermine health	The risk factors that undermine health
In terms of **whose** health, the focus is on...	The community as a whole	A particular constituent population (e.g., tenants, students, patients, or employees)
Cross-sector collaboration is viewed as...	Valuable, needed, and "natural," given different sectors' many overlapping functions and goals	Inevitably strained and difficult, given that different sectors are fundamentally distinct from one another and occupy different worlds (housing and education) A type of business transaction, in which each party gives something up and receives something in return (business)

www.phrases.org   The PHRASES Toolkit was developed in partnership with

Figure 1.1 Gaps at a Glance.

Reprinted from phrases.org/gaps-at-a-glance at https://www.phrases.org/wp-content/uploads/2020/06/Aspen-PHRASES-GapsAtAGlance-v2-MEL.pdf.

Gaps in Understanding	Experts in public health	Leaders in other sectors (*Housing, education, health systems, and business)*
The best **strategists** for cross-sector collaborations are believed to be...	Public health professionals	Health systems professionals (health systems)
Successful partnerships are considered the result of...	Institutional support	Individual leadership, and natural cooperation that grows out of shared values
Collaboration on **data-management and data-sharing** is viewed as...	Essential, and best coordinated by public health professionals with the required expertise	Valuable, in theory, though not easily implemented in practice
Public health professionals are understood to be...	Broadly skilled professionals with a "big picture" understanding of health and the ability to think innovatively about key issues in other sectors	Lacking in the necessary skills, orientation, and incentives to contribute meaningfully to the work of other sectors

*Where no sector is mentioned by name in a particular row, the way of thinking described is common to all four sectors

Interested in taking a deeper dive into the research findings?

These key gaps in understanding were identified based on interviews and peer discourse sessions from leaders and professionals in housing, education, business and health systems through research conducted by the FrameWorks Institute for the PHRASES project.

Read the full Map the Gaps **report by the FrameWorks Institute at** phrases.org.

Figure 1.1 Continued.

Health as full life versus health as absence of illness

When asked to define health, leaders in housing, education, and health systems often provided an expert-like definition, *explicitly* explaining that health is more than the absence of illness. They argued that health allows people to move forward in life, seize opportunities, and achieve goals. However, when discussing health indirectly, participants often *implicitly* defined health as the absence of illness or the default state of the body and the mind before the inevitable accumulation of pathologies and dysfunctions over time. Participants from the business sector relied primarily on the "absence of illness" model to define, and to talk about, health.

Health is medical

Many professionals associate health with medical care. They understand health deeply and implicitly as a medical issue, which places the health care system and health insurance at the forefront of their thinking. Some interviewees talked about the role of public health in providing preventive and curative health care to communities—specifically to underserved individuals. When they talked about it in this way, they typically thought about public health as a function—caring for the health of the public—rather than as an organized field of practice, and they assumed that this function was performed by the health care sector. Business participants often associated the phrase "public health" not simply with the *function* of caring for the health of the public but with the *concept* of a "government-run health care system."

Public health is not top-of-mind

When asked to define the term "public health," many participants initially were surprised and baffled. They had a hard time defining the concept and the field and needed time to articulate what they knew about public health. Leaders and professionals in housing, education, business, and health systems associate the field of public health with a narrow set of traditional functions related to preventing disease and protecting health and generally do not recognize its value as an effective partner. These perceptions undermine the willingness of these sectors to collaborate with public health, when possible, and the desire to come together to shift institutions and policy to better support and facilitate collaborations.

> RESEARCHER: When I say public health, how would you define what that is?
>
> HOUSING SECTOR LEADER: Wow. How would I explain public health? I don't know. I feel like you stumped me.

The Department of Health cultural model

Because they think about public health using a "Department of Health" model, leaders and professionals from other sectors associate public health with health departments and a traditional set of prevention and protection functions. Immunization campaigns, environmental inspections, and awareness campaigns about healthy behaviors were especially salient for participants. Business participants—especially those working in hospitality or construction—placed a strong emphasis on public health's regulatory functions and on safety inspections, which was often the only way that they saw public health and government health departments interacting with their work.

> EDUCATION SECTOR LEADER: How do educators feel about public health people? This is kind of the same as any government agency. Schools are very used to people coming in and saying, "We're here to help," but many of those same agencies also have some regulatory role. . . . The Department of Public Health can come in and shut you down if you have rodents.

Negative stereotypes of public health: Siloed and "book smart"

Leaders from other sectors reasoned that public health is heavily bureaucratic and territorial and that while public health professionals could, in theory, provide a wealth of resources and information to other sectors, in practice they lack the necessary orientation and incentives to convene cross-sector collaborations. Public health professionals are also widely assumed to be impractical researchers, not practical problem-solvers; their findings are perceived as too abstract to be actionable, and they are seen as not understanding the realities of business.

> EDUCATION SECTOR LEADER: If we look at these fields as being siloed, I think that's part of the problem. Public health and public education, you know, should be connected fields. Public health, public education, and public safety should be connected. Oftentimes, they're siloed. And so

we only talk when there's pressure, or we only talk when it's a situation that gets out of hand.

HOUSING SECTOR LEADER: One of the things we've found, especially with public health, is that they don't understand the difference between funding and finance. So they're very interested in funding, which is spending and programmatic, as opposed to thinking about interventions like housing, which require financing. . . . They don't have enough expertise about community development or finance or economics to insert themselves into those projects in ways that are very common or very effective.

HEALTH SYSTEMS SECTOR LEADER: Our relationship is with [redacted] University, in which there is a whole school of public health. We work with the academic researchers who are there, who, in fact, gather data, analyze the data, and opine as to what it is they think is affecting a community. That's helpful, but certainly not necessarily as instructive as getting down into the how-to-do-it execution phase.

How leaders understand the role of health in their work is sector-specific

When sector leaders reason about their own work, they have well-established ways of thinking about the goals of their sectors and how health interacts with them. Each of the following models is therefore specific to a single sector.

- Housing leaders think that housing is the first basic need and must be satisfied before other needs (employment, food, etc.) can be effectively addressed. As a result, they primarily understand health as an *outcome* of their work; ensuring decent housing, in other words, is a way to improve health.

• Education leaders argue that health is a necessary *input* for their work. They advocate for a "whole child" perspective that considers the social, emotional, and cognitive development of each student. Therefore, education leaders understand health—both mental and physical—as a prerequisite for effective learning.

• Business leaders assume that health is either a selling point (to attract customers and qualified employees) or a means to increase the bottom line by saving health care costs and reducing absenteeism.

• Health systems leaders think about their work in the context of the sector's transition toward population health management: promoting health by moving beyond traditional health care and fostering community conditions that keep more patients healthier at a lower cost.

Cross-sector collaborations are transactions

Leaders in housing and education, who think their sectors suffer from a chronic lack of financial and other resources, often reasoned that successful cross-sector collaborations require all parties to be able to easily identify the costs and gains of collaborations.

By and large, business participants were unfamiliar with the concept of cross-sector collaborations beyond those that involve business transactions with clients or customers, or contractual collaborations with people from other industries. At a fundamental level, they assumed that interactions with other sectors were inevitably and necessarily business transactions conducted at the level of their own firm. For business professionals, the only way to interact with other sectors in the community without "charging" for it was through charity work, which meant providing communities with a free service.

Data are descriptive, specific, and sometimes burdensome

Housing, education, and health systems leaders have many ways of thinking about data, some of which likely could be leveraged to highlight the value of collaborating with the field of public health (Figure 1.2).

- Data play a descriptive, not predictive, role in the work of sector leaders; data are used primarily to evaluate *existing* actions and programs, not to plan for *future* actions and programs.
- Data must be specific to one sector, one place, and often one organization to be relevant.
- While scientific data might be useful in confirming initial hypotheses, lived experience is a source of key evidence and insight on which sectors should rely.
- Collecting and analyzing data are sometimes perceived as burdens created by outside pressures—processes that distract from the mission of a sector or organization rather than help achieve it better and faster.

How Leaders in Other Sectors View the Value of Public Health and Cross-Sector Collaborations

What Is Health?

- Full Life
- Absence of Illness
- Health Is Medical

What Is Public Health?

- Not Top-of-Mind
- Health of the Population
- Health Care Provision
- Department of Health
- Siloed
- Book-Smart

What Shapes the Health of the Population?

- Different Definitions of Social Determinants
- Harmful Environments
- Health Individualism
- Cultural Norms of Health
- Direct Effects

How Is Health Connected to the Work of Other Sectors?

- Housing as Foundation
- Focus on the Whole Child
- Health as Selling Point
- Health Helps Bottom Line
- Population Health Management

How Do Cross-Sector Collaborations Work?

- Sectors Are Different Worlds
- Health as Big Tent
- What's In It for Me?
- Transaction
- Charity
- Individual Leadership
- "Just Do It"
- Culture of Collaboration

How Do Other Sectors Think About Data?

- Lay of the Land
- Business Forecast
- Every Community Is Different
- Lived Experience vs. Data
- Data as Burden
- Data Systems Are Complex

Figure 1.2 How Leaders in Other Sectors View the Value of Public Health and Cross-Sector Collaborations.

Reprinted from FrameWorks report "Public Health Reaching Across Sectors: Mapping the Gaps Between How Public Health Experts and Leaders in Other Sectors View Public Health and Cross-Sector Collaboration," https://www.phrases.org/map-the-gaps/wp-content/uploads/2020/07/Aspen-PHRASES-MTG-Report-2019.pdf.

Business professionals reason that data collection and analysis are the best ways to predict future trends and make informed decisions about future investments. Importantly, most data mentioned in discussions with business professionals were strictly business-related (e.g., advertising, sales, budgets).

But wait . . . there's hope

Despite the many gaps, there are important points of overlap in how public health experts and leaders from other sectors understand public health and cross-sector collaborations. These overlaps represent the common ground on which public health professionals can increase understanding of their field and what it brings to collaborations. Public health experts and other sector leaders and professionals share the following understandings:

- Health is a positive concept, and it can be proactively promoted.
- Upstream factors like housing, income, and education shape health outcomes in significant ways. (This is not true for business. The health systems sector has a particularly full understanding of how social factors create specific health challenges in the United States today, such as wide health inequalities, high obesity rates, and plateauing longevity.)
- Community health intersects with other sectors' goals in critical ways:
  - Housing deeply affects people's health.

- Good student health is a prerequisite for success in education.
- Good employee health is a means to achieve the profit goals of business.
- Health systems can affect community health beyond health care and increasingly have a financial stake in the ongoing health of their patient populations.
- Cross-sector collaborations can potentially benefit all partners involved.
- Housing complexes, schools, and health systems can function as community anchors that contribute to community health.
- Smart use of data can help sectors achieve their objectives and make a case for funding.
- Public health governmental agencies have a role to play in preventing health problems and promoting community health.

In these areas, where the thinking among leaders in other sectors is productively aligned with public health experts, public health professionals can leverage existing ideas to make the case for collaborating across sectors.

Conclusion

The findings presented in the "Map the Gaps" report indicate that public health professionals face significant challenges in communicating with professionals in other sectors. Even when sector leaders understand that upstream factors shape health outcomes in more significant ways than individual medical profiles, characteristics, and behaviors do, they don't think that cross-sector collaborations with the field of public health are the best way to address these fundamental challenges.

Other sectors' perceptions of public health and cross-sector collaborations are an obstacle to developing and maintaining partnerships with public health. These gaps in understanding profoundly limit recognition of the field's value. Yet these unproductive ways of thinking sit alongside more constructive ones, which can be leveraged and expanded to shift the thinking of sector leaders and professionals. Many sector leaders already recognize that health is tied to social and environmental context and that their goals are tied to the health of the people they serve. Public health professionals can appeal to this understanding to make a case for the mutual benefit of collaborations.

2

Communicating for Change: How We Deliver Our Ideas Matters

NAT KENDALL-TAYLOR

PUBLIC HEALTH HAS AN IMPORTANT ROLE to play in improving the health and well-being of society. The public health field has ideas and solutions that policymakers, professionals in other fields, and the public need to know about. These ideas and solutions matter. But they aren't all that matters. Ideas alone do not make change.

What public health professionals have to say is important, but so is *how* they say it.

Fifty years of social, cognitive, and behavioral science shows that how we position messages matters. The choices we make in how we communicate information can be the difference between an idea that cuts through and changes the conversation and one that gets swallowed up, bounces back, or is rejected outright. This is what the science of framing is all about.

Nat Kendall-Taylor, *Communicating for Change* In: *Talking Health.* Edited by: Mark R. Miller, Brian C. Castrucci, Rachel Locke, Julia Haskins, and Grace A. Castillo, Oxford University Press. © de Beaumont Foundation 2022. DOI: 10.1093/oso/9780197528464.003.0003

What is framing?

Framing refers to the choices we make in how we position information and the effects of these choices on perception and behavior—how people think, feel, and act. Sometimes these choices are small and seemingly inconsequential, such as the pronouns we use—whether we say "us and them" or "we." They can also be about the data we present, to make a point, or the values we endorse, to make a case for why an issue matters. These choices matter, and sometimes they matter a great deal.

COVID-19 is a case in point. The choices made in positioning messages had life-or-death consequences in terms of response, priorities, and the future of our country and its public health systems—whether those choices were about the application of labels such as "vulnerable" to whole groups of people and the othering effects of this labeling, or the appeals to social responsibility and use of historical exemplars to motivate collective action.

Frames take a variety of forms. *Values*[1] are one type of frame that helps people connect with an issue and see why it matters. Research points to differences in the way people think about issues and support solutions, based on the way that messages are presented through various values frames. *Examples* are another type of frame that can be used to show the importance of an issue, illustrate how it works, and shape thinking about what needs to be done. Different examples confer different meaning and have different effects in shaping people's thinking and actions. The Great Depression and the New Deal are examples that prime a sense of the importance of government action and responsibility following difficult times, of the need for solidarity, and of the power of public policy to improve the lives of Americans. Many people believe that the COVID-19 pandemic will serve as an important historical example going forward, although the precise meaning this example will carry and what it will be used to exemplify remain to be determined. *Metaphors* also are a powerful type of frame, channeling people's thinking about how an issue works and what should be done to address it. *Messengers* are important frames that shape how people understand issues and what they do as a result. There are other types of frames that affect thinking and behavior—from the verbs we use and how they imply or deny agency, to the way that data are presented. Even what we leave unsaid is a framing choice.

These choices, large and small, are powerful in determining what happens when we provide people with information.

Why does framing matter?

Understanding is frame-dependent

Framing theory and research tell us that the words and images we use to communicate are not inconsequential adornments but rather determine whether our communications do what we want them to. The way we position a message can determine whether it improves understanding of the ideas we want to get across, persuades people to act, or increases support for solutions.

Following are three brief examples that show what framing can do and why frames matter.

In a seminal study from 2004,[2] a representative sample of Americans received the same basic information about a political rally scheduled by a hate group. Half the people in the sample were told that the rally was about the "importance of free speech." The second half was told it was about "potential danger." Participants were then asked the same series of questions designed to determine whether they supported allowing the hate group to hold the rally. People who were asked to think about the importance of free speech were more than twice as likely to support the rally than those who read the same information presented through the lens of potential danger. The information was the same, but the way it was framed shaped people's thinking in a significant way.

In a study designed to see how different ways of presenting information about child mental health affects support for public policies,[3] a representative sample of Americans read about a fictitious program that provided support to children and their families. Study participants were randomly assigned to one of three groups. Those assigned to the first group—the control group—read the program description, without any intentional framing. Those in the second group read the same information, but it was introduced with an appeal to the value of future progress and prosperity—making the point that supporting children's mental health is important to the future success and progress of our country. Those in the third group read the same basic program information, but instead of being primed to think about future progress and prosperity, they were asked to think about the value of vulnerability—the idea that children are among the most vulnerable members of society and deserve our help, empathy, and compassion. All participants then indicated their level of support for a set of evidence-based child mental health policies. Those whose description was framed with the value of future progress and prosperity were more than twice as supportive of the policies as those who were asked to think about vulnerability. The framing of the program affected people's thinking and support for solutions.

Finally, in a study exploring public support for environmental health work,[4] a nationally representative sample was split into groups. Some participants were randomly assigned to a control group in which they read no message, while others read passages that asked them to think about environmental health through the lens of a specific value. All participants were then asked about the level of funding they thought was appropriate for environmental health work and about their support for particular environmental health policies advocated by those in the field. The study found that participants who read about the idea that "no matter where you live, you should have access to environmental health services" were more than five times more supportive of increasing funding for environmental health services than those who were presented with a message about "the importance of preventing environmental health problems."

There are numerous other examples that show how information presentation affects thinking and shapes solutions support. Examples of these frame effects were particularly rife in 2020 during the COVID-19 pandemic. COVID-19 made it clear that understanding is frame-dependent—whether it was calling the pandemic the "Chinese virus," which led to the incitement of racism and racist actions against Asian American communities (and other groups), or referring to sound and sensible public health measures as "draconian," which increased information resistance and dissuaded adherence to recommendations.

Framing is key to social and policy change

While it is well documented that the choices we make in how we communicate matter, the way that framing can help advance the field and practice of public health has received less attention.

Increasing funding for public health and implementing policies that are essential to create population health will require public understanding of and support for the field and its work. Public support is what creates space for and pressure on decision makers to make change and what prevents them from taking back ground that already has been gained. Because the way information is framed has the power to increase or decrease understanding and support, and to boost or diminish willingness to act, framing is a vital part of creating the changes the field is working for. Public health cannot ignore the power of framing and must utilize this tool to help make the changes necessary for the field to realize its potential and build a healthy society.

There is a difference between what we say and what others hear and think

Anyone who has communicated information (that is, everyone) has, at one time or another, been caught in a precarious situation: The message they thought would resonate and move someone's thinking misses the mark. Either it falls flat, failing to get people to stop and take note, or it engages people but moves them in an unintended direction. We deliver a public address that we think champions the importance of science, evidence, and research, only to have people come back to us questioning the motives of researchers, the relativeness of data, and the basic premise of the scientific process. We think we have just delivered a brilliant call to action about the difficulty of parenting and the need for greater public support for families, only to have people walk away even more convinced that parents need to make better decisions, and that ultimately there isn't anything we as a society can do to improve their parenting or their child's development. We write an article or blog post about all the things the field of public health does to support society and the range of organizations engaged in this work, only to have people leave negative comments about federal agencies. We talk with a relative about the disproportionate impact of COVID-19 on communities of color, aiming to shed light on the structural causes of such disparities, only to have our loved one respond with a statement about the unfortunate nature of decisions that people of certain groups make and their deficient values or "culture."

These are examples of the "backfire" effect: We think we are communicating one thing but discover that our audience is taking away something different. In some cases, the takeaway is entirely at odds with what we intended to communicate. These experiences are perplexing, and they inhibit our ability to communicate effectively. But we can understand what is going on here and why. We can see—and even predict—when these misinterpretations will occur.

The "you say/they think" phenomenon is the result of culture and the way it stands between everything that we say and everything that people take from our messages. Culture in this context doesn't mean what is typically associated with the field of anthropology—visible behaviors, explicit beliefs, or material artifacts and symbols. Instead, it means *culture in mind.* Culture in mind is the idea that, in addition to its material and conscious components, culture exists as a set of shared mental models and patterns of reasoning that we use, without being aware of them, to make sense of information. Psychological anthropologists call this facet of culture "cultural models." Cultural models are the assumptions and patterns of reasonings that we unknowingly apply when presented with information and processing it. Cultural models inform our understanding of any message and what we do as a result. They explain how we can aim a message in one direction only to have it boomerang back at us.

We see the backfire effect frequently in our work at the FrameWorks Institute. For example, when an organization is trying to communicate about the detrimental effects of severe and chronic stress in early childhood, the messages often are interpreted in counterintuitive ways. Many people respond to messages that early adversity can derail development with strong affirmations of the importance of stress in building character and driving positive growth and development. This may seem confusing if you're the communicator caught in this lost-in-translation moment. But this is an example of a cultural model in action. When primed to consider the effects of stress, many Americans think of the aphorism "what doesn't kill you makes you stronger." They use this assumption to process information about stress. Because the message about the detrimental effects of stress contains a frame (stress) that cues culture in mind ("what doesn't kill you . . ."), the resulting perspective ends up in opposition to the message and its intent. The intention of the message is out of alignment with its effect.

Public health professionals also experience the backfire effect. They talk about the systems, structures, and resources that shape health and the importance of public health in promoting conditions that advance positive health at a population level. But because they are priming people's culture in mind about health, they get responses that focus on individuals, behaviors, and disease—ideas that are, in many ways, in opposition to the ideas we are trying to advance. FrameWorks calls this "health individualism." Health individualism is the assumption that health outcomes are the exclusive and narrow result of an individual's choices, decisions, and will. This way of thinking makes messages about systems, populations, and structures boomerang and backfire. When we talk about systems, people think about individual behaviors and choices. And yelling louder about systems and populations only makes the situation worse. It's not the ideas that are wrong; it's the way they are presented—the way they are framed.

Communicators need to understand the culture in mind they are communicating into and position messages intentionally in relation to these understandings. Being an expert communicator means becoming an expert in the culture that will be used to process our messages.

The good news is that we can understand culture in mind. When we do, we can make more-informed decisions and position our messages for better effect. This practice of seeing culture is at the root of strategic framing.

How can we frame more strategically?

In FrameWorks' research, we've learned three things about strategic framing that can help public health communicators better position their messages, discussed next.

1. Repeating what we want people to forget doesn't shift thinking.

"Logical" and "effective" don't always line up when it comes to communicating about public health issues. When presented with a misperception, logic tells us to take it on, point out why it is incorrect, and then move to the truth. Research on childhood vaccinations and flu vaccines show that this debunking approach fails to correct misperceptions, and in some cases may actually strengthen them. This effect has also been visible during the COVID-19 pandemic, in that many people tried to correct misperceptions about vaccines, inadvertently repeating—and strengthening—myths in their attempts to refute them.

Thinking about framing can help us understand why the debunking approach is ineffective and identify a more productive tack for correcting misperceptions. The logic of the debunking strategy is that, once activated, the faulty belief can be taken on, disproven, and then replaced with an alternative idea that usually will be more abstract and less familiar. Unfortunately, this is not how our cognitive system works. Once a person is reminded of the existing belief, that belief only grows stronger. Once our existing understanding has been primed, we feel like we know the answer and we suspend more effortful thinking. The new information that follows the evocation of the existing misperception falls on deaf ears. The misperception is left undisturbed and even strengthened by getting another chance to activate and shape thinking. Framing research tells us that repeating the thing we want people to forget is an ineffective strategy for correcting misperceptions.

Understanding why this strategy doesn't work informs our thinking about what we should do instead. If we lead with and explain the position that we want to advance, we have a better chance of shifting and correcting misperceptions. Correcting misperceptions is about advancing the idea that we want to build up in people's thinking. Framing messages in ways that lead with and repeat the idea that we want to advance is more effective than giving a misperception more air, exercise, and room to breathe.

2. Focusing on problems doesn't lead people to solutions.

Balancing urgency with efficacy is key in creating engaging and persuasive communications. Public health professionals tend to focus their messages on problems and hit hard on urgency. The thinking behind this approach is that if people can see how dire a particular problem is, they will be motivated to engage to address the problem. But messages that start and end with crisis, emergency, and urgency don't actually have this effect. In fact, they can do the opposite—make people feel fatalistic and more likely to disengage. Messages that focus on problems can give people a sense of the gravity of the problem, but that alone isn't enough to change thinking and motivate action. By itself, a really heavy problem is just that. Crisis doesn't translate into action.

This isn't to say that the gravity that comes from urgency doesn't matter. It does, but it needs help from a second vital element—efficacy. Efficacy is the sense that there are things that can be done to remediate and address an issue or situation. We can build efficacy by sharing examples of solutions with an explanation about how they can fix the problem, or by adopting a tone that conveys the sense that solutions are possible. When we add a dose of efficacy to the grip of urgency, we get effective communications and powerful messages.

Framing our messages to balance urgency and efficacy can help move an audience's thinking and motivate action.

3. Explanation is powerful.

The way we choose to frame our messages can make people smarter about how issues work. When people better under-stand how an issue works, they become more able to identify effective solutions and more confident in their support for actions. Explanation is a powerful part of effective framing.

Understanding matters, and you can buttress it by using a range of techniques—such as examples or arguments that care-fully explain how determinants cause outcomes. Metaphors are particularly effective explanatory tools.

Metaphors work by taking something familiar—the "source domain"—and comparing it with something less familiar—the "target domain"—which allows people to see something un-familiar in a familiar light and thus arrive at a better under-standing of how it works. Carefully developed metaphors can draw on things that people already understand and help them make sense of something less familiar. If similarities between the source and the target domains are carefully mapped and tested, metaphors can be used to increase understanding of otherwise complex or confusing topics.

For example, if the concept of executive function from the science of early childhood were described as the "brain's air traffic control system," you would start to understand some of the key concepts from the science of executive function. This metaphor would allow you to develop a concept of the phe-nomenon that closely resembles the scientific understanding. You would get smarter in a quick and immediate way. You would see that executive function must be about the ability to hold and coordinate multiple things in mind at once. You'd get that it must be about carefully sequencing and managing demands. And you could see that it must entail the need to be flexible and adapt to changing situations and challenges.

Similarly, if you were told that brains are built like a house, you could draw on your understandings of structures and construction to understand that what happens early in brain development must be important for everything that follows. You could see that there must be a sequence and an order to the process of developing "brain architecture" and that timing matters. The metaphor could increase your understanding that what happens early affects what comes later—all through just a few words required to set the metaphor.

Explanatory tools like metaphors increase understanding of how an issue works. And with this, people can recognize and support solutions and actions necessary to improve outcomes. When applied to public health, these explanatory tools can be used to channel attention toward specific solutions (the need for better preventive systems, for example) and away from others (the perception that health is a matter of individual choices and decisions).

Conclusion

Framing research is clear: How you position your messages and present your ideas can increase support for public health and collaboration across sectors. On the other hand, if you are not deliberate about your framing, your message can backfire by fomenting misunderstandings of public health and increasing resistance to collaboration among those you need as partners.

Focusing on the ideas you want to communicate (and not repeating misperceptions), including a robust sense of both urgency and efficacy, and making sure that your communications explain fundamental principles of public health are essential to ensuring that you are communicating effectively and driving action. These ideas are vital parts of effective public health practice and core skills for practitioners to learn and deploy.

If understanding is frame-dependent, then increasing support for public health requires that you be attentive to the way you frame your messages. This book is designed to help you do this work—to frame your information in ways that cut through, get heard, shift thinking, and change hearts and minds.

3

Winning Words and Strategic Stories: Building Public Support for Public Health

DOUG HATTAWAY AND ERIC ZIMMERMANN

ON A FALL EVENING IN 2019, six residents of San Jose, California, filed into a nondescript market research facility, seated themselves around a conference room table, and eyed with curiosity the double-sided mirror at the far end of the room.

In the mirror's reflection, they saw a diverse group—men and women; young and old; Black, white, Latino, and Asian American. The group included Democrats, Independents, and Republicans, but they shared one thing in common: They were among the country's most active citizens. These focus group participants had been selected for their level of civic engagement: They voted regularly, volunteered in their communities, followed the news, and shared information on social media about issues they consider important. We hoped that their

Doug Hattaway and Eric Zimmermann, *Winning Words and Strategic Stories* In: *Talking Health*.
Edited by: Mark R. Miller, Brian C. Castrucci, Rachel Locke, Julia Haskins, and Grace A. Castillo, Oxford
University Press. © de Beaumont Foundation 2022. DOI: 10.1093/oso/9780197528464.003.0004

demonstrated interest in the world would foster a lively and thought-provoking conversation.

This was the first of several focus groups that Hattaway Communications held around the country to explore a simple but daunting issue: how to get members of the general public to understand and support public health. After an introductory icebreaker and some small talk, the moderator posed a query: "If someone tells you they work in public health, what do you think they do?"

After a long, silent pause, a middle-aged woman we'll call Susan ventured a response: "My sister works for the CDC," she said. "She works for some division, and it's all the bureaucrats— the pencil pushers who are making all these dumb laws."

That dismissive response reflects something important about the way our brains process information: How we perceive the individuals who are part of a field determines what we think of the field itself. Susan thinks first of "bureaucrats" or "pencil pushers," so it follows that she thinks workers in public health make "dumb laws."

Equally important is what's missing from Susan's answer: She sees no connection between public health and the life she wants to lead. Contrast Susan's answer with her fellow participants' vivid and personal thoughts when asked what "being healthy" means:

"Being healthy means meeting your desired lifestyle. So, if you like working in the yard, if you can't physically do that, then by definition you wouldn't be healthy."

"Healthy is feeling good in the skin you're in."

"Technically, healthy means absence of disease; however, it's a lot broader than that, and includes being balanced in mental, physical, and spiritual well-being."

The gap between people's vague perceptions of public health and their deeply held beliefs about their personal health has frustrated public health professionals for generations. But the fault doesn't lie entirely with the audience. For people to see the impact of public health, they need to see *themselves* in public health. They need to connect public health and their own health, and they need to see how the goals of public health are consistent with the aspirations they have for their own lives. That's what makes a topic relevant and meaningful and encourages people to stop and think about it. Making those connections is a task that falls to public health professionals— and the language and stories they use to explain their work.

Words matter: Make them winning words

It may seem like a truism that when it comes to communication, words matter. But too often we take for granted how much language influences the way we process information and perceive the world.

Consider the words and phrases our focus group participants used when discussing their personal health: "You like working in the yard" and "Feeling good in the skin you're in." These descriptions have two things in common. First, they're vivid: You can visualize someone "working in the yard," and "the skin you're in" is a familiar representation of a person's relationship with their own body. Language that creates visual images in people's minds is easier to understand and remember. It also activates the visual cortex of the brain along with the language center. Our brains literally are more engaged when we process vivid language.

Second, both quotes describe an emotion: "You like working" suggests fulfillment, and "Feeling good" obviously suggests contentment and pleasure. Emotion works with cognition to help us process information. Our emotions cue us to focus on what's important to us, think about it, and remember it. If language creates an emotional response, we're more likely to pay attention and consider the ideas meaningful. It's not surprising that people can immediately conjure vivid and emotional language when describing a topic as personal as their own health.

Now consider the language Susan used to discuss public health: "some division," "bureaucrats," "dumb laws." This is abstract language, suggesting that Susan can't visualize what public health means in practice. This probably isn't her fault: Public health messengers often use technical jargon that is almost impossible for non-experts to understand, let alone visualize. Jargon develops within communities of experts who all speak the same language. Linguists call these "discourse communities." Within those communities, everyone is on the same page, and jargon serves as a convenient shorthand to speed up communication. But more often than not, that jargon finds its way into communication with broader audiences. When that happens, jargon is no longer helpful. In fact, it prevents your audience from understanding what you're saying. To them, you're speaking a foreign language.

The job of public health professionals, educators, and communicators is to frame public health with language that helps non-experts visualize its impact on their lives. In focus groups, we tested messages that used simple, vivid language to describe the need for public health. One statement, for example, read, "Threats to our health can come from all kinds of places—the food we eat, the water we drink, and the air we breathe." We found that respondents immediately were able to paint a picture of how public health related to their lives:

> "Where I live, they're doing a lot of home building, and they actually just shut it down recently because they weren't watering down the dirt enough, and so that's why that kind of related to me—'the air we breathe.' "

Think about the visual imagery you'd like people to associate with your work. It could be a physical place ("safe neighborhoods"), a tangible object ("the food we eat"), or a personal experience ("hugging your family"). Use this language to frame conversations about your work—like the intentionally vivid descriptions of public health given below—and you'll have taken the first step toward more motivating communications.

From winning words to strategic stories

Once we've translated abstract words, we're faced with the daunting task of translating complex ideas. Public health professionals work within a complicated web of laws, systems, and data, and we need our audience to grasp how it all connects to their lives. That understanding starts with stories.

Today, storytelling is the vogue in management and communications circles, but it's anything but a fad. From the time humans developed the capacity for language, our brains have evolved to understand the world through stories—precisely because stories have so many qualities that help us understand the complex world. Most notably, stories provide a shortcut for understanding cause-and-effect relationships. From birth, identifying these relationships is one of our primary cognitive tasks. It's why toddlers never get tired of asking, "Why?"

Stories answer the "why" by turning multifaceted events into simple cause-and-effect relationships, complete with characters we can envision. As Nobel Prize–winning psychologist Daniel Kahneman writes in his bestselling book, *Thinking Fast and Slow,* "The mind . . . appears to have a special aptitude for the construction and interpretation of stories about active agents, who have personalities, habits, and abilities." Stories are especially useful when a situation is complex or the cause of a problem is hard to pin down—like in public health. Instead of abstract ideas, trends, or figures, stories introduce the people affected by the problem, those who caused the problem, and those with the power to create change.

The primary purpose of public health storytelling isn't artistic—it's strategic. Strategic storytelling is intended to motivate a specific group of people—your audience—to take specific actions. To do that, you need to shape your stories to communicate specific ideas that are likely to motivate the audience. Our focus group discussions were designed to identify those motivating ideas and help us create a conceptual framework for public health professionals to use in crafting stories that resonate with the general public. To learn more about that research effort and the insights we gained, see the public health communications toolkit included in PHRASES (Public Health Reaching Across Sectors; see Chapter 4).

Below are four key elements of a strategic story for public health. Each includes language informed by our focus groups that tells the story of public health as a field, along with questions you can use to adapt the framework to create your own story about a specific public health situation.

1. **People: Describe public health professionals in terms that will resonate with your audience.** An effective story starts with putting people in the picture. But you need to do so in a strategic way. To replace the aloof "pencil pushers" Susan imagines, describe the expertise that public health professionals bring to their work and their involvement in the communities they serve.

   Public health experts are trained to diagnose the health of a community. They listen to people who know their community best and draw on science and data to recognize patterns and problems.

   Tell your story: Who do you work with? Describe your public health colleagues, including their expertise and how they work with and listen to the communities they serve.

2. **Goals: Connect the goals of public health to the aspirations people have for their own lives.** This seems straightforward—everyone wants to lead a

healthy life, and that's what public health helps them do. But stating that a public health professional is going to "keep you healthy" can rob people of their sense of agency—and trigger skepticism. Instead, use concrete examples like air, food, and water to help people visualize how public health prevents disease and injury—enabling them to make their own healthy choices.

Public health is designed to prevent each of us from getting sick or injured in the first place. Clean air, pure water, safe neighborhoods, and more—it's the mission of public health to make sure our cities, communities, and country have what we need to stay healthy.

Tell your story: What is the goal of your work, and how does it keep people healthy and prevent disease or injury? Use vivid words and relatable examples.

3. **Problems: Frame the problems that public health addresses in a way that people can understand— and that sounds solvable.** Public health problems that sound too overwhelming or complex can demotivate audiences, who may feel that an issue is intractable. Describe the consequences of the problem for people's lives and, if relevant, note how health care alone is ill-equipped to address the challenge.

In the United States, we spend so much time and money on health care, but we're not getting healthier. That's because we wait to treat people until after they're sick or injured.

Tell your story: What problems stand in the way of your goal? Make the consequences of this problem clear but avoid being overly complex. If relevant, describe how traditional health care is not equipped to solve this problem.

4. **Solutions: Be specific about what public health professionals do—and how it benefits both individuals and communities.** Describe the actions public health experts take to prevent disease and injury. Go beyond laws and policies—use specific examples to explain how each action can improve an individual's health by addressing health threats before they start.

   Public health experts bring together everyone who has a role to play in their community's health—schools, businesses, government agencies, and others—to stop health threats before they start.

   Tell your story: How does your work solve the previously mentioned problems? Emphasize collaborative approaches and show how the people you serve benefit from your work.

Conclusion

Among the many lessons we've learned from the COVID-19 pandemic is how dangerous it can be to cast public health communications in a secondary, supporting role. From the outset of the pandemic, the public received mixed messages on mask wearing and confusing information about who should be tested and when. Technical debates important to experts—like whether someone with barely noticeable symptoms should be described as "asymptomatic"—leaked into the public conversation, confused people, and led some to act on false assumptions.

We have learned the hard way that even the most sound, common-sense strategies—mask wearing, regular testing, contract tracing—will fail if we can't motivate people to participate. In other words, the language we use and the stories we tell are just as important as the data we mine and the studies we publish.

But we've also learned that health communication isn't a task solely for public health professionals. Hospital administrators, school principals, property managers, airline CEOs, small-business owners, and more have all been enlisted as public health communicators. They're tasked not only with making their facilities safe but with explaining their strategies to patients, customers, students, and employees. If cross-sector collaboration for public health had once seemed abstract, it is now all too real.

Communicating more effectively means changing longstanding habits—and habit change is hard. To begin, employ the resources in front of you. The PHRASES tools (see Chapter 4) and other insights shared in this book can equip public health professionals with the information they need to become more effective communicators—and to better advance the mission of public health.

Next, don't feel the need to have all the answers, but push yourself to ask the right questions. For example, public health experts would be thrilled if leaders in other sectors asked: "There's probably evidence on how this decision affects people's health—what do the data say?" Public health experts should similarly ask themselves, "There's probably evidence on the best way to communicate this—what do the data say?"

Finally, ask for help. If you have communications staff on your team, they almost certainly have encountered the same challenge you're facing, have tried different solutions, and can tell you what works best. We guarantee they'll be thrilled you asked.

Part II
Tools and Perspectives

4

Tools: Effective Messaging and Storytelling for Public Health

MARK R. MILLER AND RACHEL LOCKE

THE TOOLS PROVIDED HERE WERE DEVELOPED as part of the PHRASES (Public Health Reaching Across Sectors) initiative to help public health professionals and advocates communicate more effectively about the value of public health. These tools can be applied to nearly any type of health communication. This section summarizes the main tools and recommendations developed through PHRASES; additional detail and other resources can be found at www.phra ses.org.

The tools are based on research by the FrameWorks Institute, a nonprofit research organization that helps mission-driven organizations build public will for progressive change, and Hattaway Communications, a strategic communications firm that uses the power of strategy, science, and storytelling to improve impact. The FrameWorks Institute conducted research with four key sectors—housing, education, business,

Mark R. Miller and Rachel Locke, *Tools* In: *Talking Health.* Edited by: Mark R. Miller, Brian C. Castrucci, Rachel Locke, Julia Haskins, and Grace A. Castillo, Oxford University Press. © de Beaumont Foundation 2022. DOI: 10.1093/oso/9780197528464.003.0005 and health systems—and produced a "Map the Gaps" report, a Strategic Framing Brief, and framing recommendations and tools. Hattaway Communications translated this sector-specific research and their own research into tools for communicating to general audiences, as well as storytelling and collaboration tools.

Frame elements

Frames are sets of choices we make when we present information—what to emphasize, how to explain ourselves, and what to leave unsaid. A *frame element* is a communications device that alters the presentation (but not the content) of a message—such as a metaphor that helps clarify a concept, a cultural value or shared principle that signals broad relevance, or a particular tone that the messenger adopts (see "Tapping into the power of metaphors," below).

Every communication involves many different frame elements, although they aren't always chosen strategically. The following frame elements were designed specifically to close critical gaps in understanding between public health experts and professionals in other sectors. They were also tested in multiple settings and shown to be extremely effective.

The Value of Investment

The Value of Investment frame element (Figure 4.1) is a deeply held and widely shared commitment to using monetary and other resources effectively, with an eye toward long-term gain.

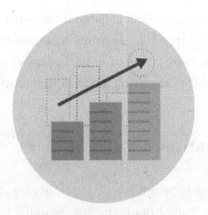

The Value of Investment

Figure 4.1 The Value of Investment.
Reprinted from phrases.org. https://www.phrases.org/tools/.

THE STORY YOU'RE TELLING

Successful organizations manage their resources carefully to align short- and long-term goals. Public health professionals want to work collaboratively with other sectors to save money in the short term whenever possible and make wise investments over the long term that support community health, increase efficiency, and reduce unnecessary costs for everyone.

TASKS THAT CAN BE ACCOMPLISHED USING THIS FRAME ELEMENT

- Orient thinking among potential partners toward the possibilities for joint endeavors that are mutually beneficial, both financially and strategically, in terms of achieving organizational objectives and goals.

- Instill confidence that collaborations with public health can achieve attainable, measurable successes.
- Extend the time frame of typical cost–benefit analyses to include multiyear considerations and increasing gains over time.

CONCEPTS AND IDEAS INCLUDED IN THIS FRAME ELEMENT

- Controlling expenses is a chief priority for all professional sectors, including public health. Working together to improve health outcomes for the entire community is an investment that pays off for everyone.
- A long-term view is required to reap the cost savings and other benefits of building a strong foundation that supports community health.

PRACTICAL APPLICATION

FrameWorks research found that broad claims made by public health professionals about the general importance and beneficial nature of collaboration are ineffective with other sectors. In fact, when they lack concrete details and specificity, such claims cause frustration and invite skepticism or even pushback. A Value of Investment appeal can protect communications against this "backfire" effect, but its ability to do so requires that messages address each of the following:

- **A clear timeline.** Knowing when the rewards of collaboration are likely to be enjoyed empowers prospective

partners to assess for themselves how they want to participate, which makes participation itself more desirable.

- **A precise accounting.** Other sectors' interest in
collaborating with public health increases with the level of
detail they are provided—both about the initial investment
of resources that a particular initiative requires and about
the projected recuperations or other measurable outcomes
it is expected to produce.

- **A dollar figure.** While the full benefits of collaboration
may not translate onto a balance sheet, fiscal arguments
are uniquely enticing for many sector professionals—most
notably those in business. Whenever monetary advantages
can be identified and itemized, explicit mention of them
will add efficacy and expedience to a collaboration-focused
communication.

GPS Navigation

GPS Navigation (Figure 4.2) is a metaphor for how the field of
public health engages data to support the work of other sectors
in innovative and forward-thinking ways.

THE STORY YOU'RE TELLING

GPS is a powerful tool for visualizing and navigating complex
terrain, and public health professionals serve this function,
too. We draw on a wealth of data to chart routes from where
we are as a community to where we want to be. Most of all, we
put our data expertise to work to drive positive outcomes and
move needed solutions forward.

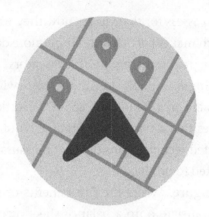

GPS Navigation

Figure 4.2 GPS Navigation.
Reprinted from phrases.org. https://www.phrases.org/tools/.

TASKS THAT CAN BE ACCOMPLISHED USING THIS FRAME ELEMENT

- Foster greater understanding of data's problem-solving power beyond its monitoring and tracking functions.
- Build awareness among professionals in other sectors about the value and extent of public health's data expertise.
- Illustrate for potential partners how public health data and public health professionals' data skills can be harnessed to enhance the work they do.

CONCEPTS AND IDEAS INCLUDED IN THIS FRAME ELEMENT

- Careful and informed planning is required to successfully navigate the complex terrain of community health.

- Data are an essential tool—not only for visualizing the landscape but for mapping a range of possible routes that lead from point A to point B.
- Expertise is required to seek out, sort, and make sense of relevant data—and public health professionals have the necessary skills.
- Like GPS, public health's data expertise is a practical and versatile instrument. It provides information and generates recommendations, based on user input, but doesn't give commands or take control.
- Public health's proficiency with data offers other sectors access to a wealth of practical knowledge about intersecting priorities, important landmarks, optional shortcuts, and potential roadblocks that lie ahead.
- Forward-thinking ingenuity and social innovation are enabled by public health's data expertise. It functions like an infinitely adaptable device—accounting for numerous dynamic factors, enabling interactive step-by-step course-plotting, troubleshooting unexpected conditions, and maneuvering through traffic jams as needed to rev up community health outcomes and drive positive change.

PRACTICAL APPLICATION

- Steer clear of messages that put public health professionals in the driver's seat. Other sector professionals don't necessarily want to hand over the wheel!
- Avoid describing public health's role as "giving directions."
- Be careful not to imply that public health professionals know how to pick the "best" route. It's preferable to show

how data can be used to help identify multiple routes rather than focus on any single one.

Foundation of Community Health

Foundation of Community Health (Figure 4.3) is a metaphor for how the health of a community is supported by the work of professionals in many different sectors.

THE STORY YOU'RE TELLING

The health of our community is like a building—it depends on a strong and stable foundation. Things like quality education, safe and affordable housing, access to health care, and employment opportunities structure positive health outcomes for

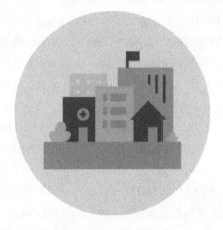

Foundation of Community Health

Figure 4.3 Foundation of Community Health.
Reprinted from phrases.org. https://www.phrases.org/tools/.

everyone in important ways. As public health professionals, it's our mission to build thriving communities, so we work closely with many other sectors to assemble a solid foundation that supports long-lasting good health for us all.

TASKS THAT CAN BE ACCOMPLISHED USING THIS FRAME ELEMENT

- Enhance understanding among professionals in other sectors of the social determinants of health.
- Help other sectors appreciate that positive health outcomes should be actively supported, beyond simply avoiding negative health outcomes.
- Encourage other sectors to see that community health is about much more than ensuring that individuals make healthy lifestyle choices and have access to health care—it depends on reliable structures and strong social systems that we all help to build.

CONCEPTS AND IDEAS INCLUDED IN THIS FRAME ELEMENT

- Good health is much more than just the absence of illness. It is the overall state of well-being for individuals and communities.
- Health must be actively constructed by promoting protective factors and creating positive conditions. It cannot be optimally achieved only by treating sickness and eliminating threats.
- It's not only individuals who experience health outcomes—entire communities do, too. By strengthening supports for

everyone, we can improve the health of the community as a whole.

- Laying the groundwork for good health is a task that requires an all-hands-on-deck approach. All skill sets, all people, and all communities are therefore assets in this collective endeavor. (They should never be mistaken for problems that need to be "fixed.")
- Like any construction project, building community health requires careful planning, information-sharing, teamwork, and many skilled contributions. Ensuring the success of the project, through support and coordination, is the mission of public health.

PRACTICAL APPLICATIONS

- Avoid placing public health in a leadership role. When applying the Foundation of Community Health metaphor, it's best to avoid depicting public health professionals as the "foremen/forewomen" or "architects." Doing so may seem presumptuous to professionals in other sectors—especially if they see themselves as leaders in the health sphere.
- Use the metaphor to explain the social determinants of health framework. It is not easy for non-experts to grasp. Rather than simply listing social determinants and asserting their importance, public health professionals should use the metaphor to explain how social factors support or undermine health.
- Instead of the phrase "social determinants of health," consider describing the relevant factors or conditions in terms

of "the foundations of health" or "the foundations of community health." This alternative language is easier for people outside of public health to understand and focuses attention on the importance of working together to improve health outcomes for everyone.

Framing recommendations

1. Demonstrate familiarity with the sectors you wish to engage

Framing can help enhance the credibility of the public health field and earn another sector's trust by demonstrating knowledge of that sector's inner workings and diverse elements and, where appropriate, addressing key internal distinctions that exist. Most of all, avoid talking about "the housing sector" or "the business sector" as a whole, and instead refer to the particular subgroups within that sector you aim to reach.

2. Explain the social determinants of health using the Foundation of Community Health metaphor

Framing can help other sectors understand health in more proactive, holistic, and structural terms. The Foundation of Community Health metaphor conveys that the many different issues tied to a community's health are also connected to one another, which helps professionals in all sectors to see that they must work together to achieve shared success.

3. Illustrate how the field of public health is transforming to meet twenty-first century needs

Framing can help alleviate some of the confusion for other sectors by acknowledging that, historically, public health served a narrower function but that it has evolved and is still transforming. Highlight where the field is going by referring to specific attributes of Public Health 3.0, and make clear that it is adopting innovative approaches that are increasingly responsive to the needs of an interconnected and modern world.

4. Leverage allies and public health professionals working in or with other sectors as messengers

Framing can help potential collaborators focus on their commonalities rather than dwell on their differences. The trick is to let professionals with cross-sector experience do the talking. Whenever possible, feature the perspectives and firsthand accounts of practitioners whose understanding spans another sector in addition to public health.

5. Frame collaboration as empowerment

Framing can help assuage other sectors' fears of being asked to relinquish control by affirming their existing priorities and acknowledging their ongoing efforts. Likewise, conveying how public health proposes to support another sector's mission goes a long way toward helping its professionals see collaboration as an asset rather than a liability.

6. Appeal to the Value of Investment to orient thinking toward tangible long-term gains

Framing can help acknowledge other sectors' resource concerns while encouraging them to think in "bigger-picture" and longer-term ways about the benefits of community health. Whenever possible, highlight opportunities to align short-term objectives with long-term goals, and spell out any monetary or other material benefits of doing so.

7. Share vivid success stories that link cross-sector collaborations to the concrete benefits they deliver

Framing can help bring concrete evidence of the benefits of collaboration to bear. By drawing on recent and detailed success stories, involving actual initiatives by real people in identified places, communications can convincingly answer the "but how?" question that lingers in prospective collaborators' minds.

8. Foreground public health's data expertise

Framing can help establish an association between public health and data sets, as well as data analysis and proficiency. Messages that vividly exhibit public health professionals' data expertise, particularly by describing their ability to use data as a problem-solving tool, can help other sectors appreciate the utility and applicability of the field.

9. Use the GPS Navigation metaphor to explain how public health's data expertise can help other sectors move toward innovative solutions

Framing can help explain how public health's data expertise works, particularly how it can function as a flexible and adaptable tool for other sectors to engage with interactively. Effective communications illustrate that data—in the skilled hands of public health experts and with the essential input of sector professionals—can spark cutting-edge ideas, revolutionize on-the-ground practices, and implement state-of-the-art improvements.

10. Keep it positive

Framing can help motivate action and the sense of a common mission by invoking shared values, offering explanation, providing context, and detailing helpful examples. In projecting a constructive can-do attitude and positive outlook, the field of public health can advance a mobilizing vision—of safer, healthier, and more prosperous communities—that professionals in all sectors see themselves as having a role in and are inspired to help build.

Tapping into the power of metaphors

Metaphorical language—which includes metaphors, similes, analogies, and other comparisons—is a powerful tool in social change communications.

Metaphors that rely on everyday objects or experiences can help introduce unfamiliar issues or explain complex ones. This is especially helpful when we need to put a new issue on the public agenda or make sure that sound science informs policy decisions.

Metaphors can spark new associations and understandings, placing an issue in a new light and prompting people to rethink their opinions or assumptions. When we need to shift widely shared mindsets, the right metaphor can make the difference.

And because metaphors give us a new mental framework for thinking and talking about a topic, they can open up dead-end conversations and repetitive debates. Using metaphors can help us advance ideas and avoid wasting energy by rebutting talking points that halt progressive change.

Metaphors are powerful, and we can use them to build understanding and shape the conversation on social issues. But we need to use them wisely and carefully. Here are three principles for using metaphor as a tool for social change.

1. Rely on research

Metaphors can powerfully affect understanding and opinions, but sometimes they work in ways we do not expect or foresee. A metaphor highlights some things and hides others. Each comes with its own set of emphases and blind spots. We cannot reliably predict, based only on our own close-to-the-issue intuition, how large numbers of people will respond to a metaphor. The right comparison can advance our issues—but the wrong one can set us back.

We do not need to leave this to chance. The FrameWorks Institute has tested hundreds of metaphors on dozens of social issues over the years—with each freely available study typically involving multiple research methods and a sample of several thousand people. In most cases, therefore, we can use metaphors that have been tested, to make sure they faithfully represent important concepts, build understanding, and promote progressive policy preferences. On issues for which metaphors have not been tested, we can simulate their explanatory power with other techniques—like laying out cause-and-effect links or using well-crafted examples.

2. Introduce metaphors early—and explicitly

Metaphors are more effective in social-change communications than other approaches. Explanatory metaphors help people make sense of a topic. If we introduce them early, they guide how people respond to the rest of the communication.

However, we should avoid introducing distracting metaphors. For example, if we start by naming the issue—as is common in political campaigning—that may unlock all the associations that people have with a topic, such as anti-Black stereotypes associated with "welfare" or the political polarization attached to "climate change." Often, these are the very ideas we are trying to change. Reminding people of those associated beliefs makes changing mindsets and shifting thinking harder than they need to be.

If we begin by reciting the research on the topic, another common practice, people may tune out. This is especially true when we present an audience with a lengthy list of negative outcomes, leading people to conclude that the problem is too big to solve.

While avoiding the wrong metaphors and overwhelming research, we still often need to provide a context for our message.

When we do not offer a frame of reference, people fall back on frames and mindsets they have picked up elsewhere. Metaphors can help us avoid this by proactively opening channels for people to think about new ideas.

For example, many communications about adolescent development start out by acknowledging the risks associated with adolescence and the need to protect young people from danger, or they cite statistics about the number of young people who experience mental health challenges.

Instead of using this approach, it can be more productive to lead with a metaphor of adolescence as a time of exploration, when young people need to test ideas, experiment with boundaries, and be able to take and learn from safe risks. Elaborating on the metaphor offers the audience a way to replace unproductive mental pictures of young people as reckless—and adolescence as a period of danger—with a more balanced understanding of the risks and opportunities and a sense of the potential for powerful learning and development.

3. Extend metaphors over time, across contexts, and across networks

For new ways of thinking to take root, we must continuously cultivate them. This involves repeating our ideas (without sounding repetitive) and engaging others in sharing and expressing those same ideas in their own way.

Metaphors lend themselves to both consistency and creativity, so many communications professionals can use them without sounding scripted or inauthentic. The basic comparison can and should remain stable—this is how a field taps into the power of repetition. But the emphasis, the style, and even the medium or messenger can vary significantly.

A good example comes from FrameWorks' long-standing partnership with the Center on the Developing Child at Harvard University, which has led to the creation of several metaphors to translate key concepts in early childhood development. The metaphor of brain architecture has been used by a wide range of experts, including neuroscientists, policy advocates, and staff at child care centers. Brain architecture has been used as an organizing theme for university lectures, tabletop games, media interviews, public-service announcements, and interactive museum exhibits.

Sometimes communications professionals highlight the importance of having a solid foundation; other times, they use the sequencing of a construction project to help illustrate a developmental concept. Through this varied set of expressions, the early childhood field has brought the same fundamental idea (early brain development matters) to life in fresh ways again and again, across a decade. As a result, public thinking and public policy have shifted in major and measurable ways.

Conclusion

Metaphors are not only literary devices but also devices for thinking. They can put a picture in the public's mind where none existed before—and they can reshape and update our shared mental images of social issues. When we use them wisely in our social-change communications, we can amplify our impact.

"Tapping into the power of metaphors" was originally published by the FrameWorks Institute, August 2020, at: www.frameworksinstitute. org.

Communication tools: Building support for public health

The following section is adapted from "Motivating the Public to Support Public Health: A Toolkit for Communicating with Non-Experts," July 2020. Available at www.phrases.org.

The research-based language, guidance, and best practices in this section can help you start conversations with non-experts and frame public health in a way that is relevant to their lives. These tools and messages are not intended to serve as a comprehensive definition of public health or to replace other materials the field has developed. Rather, their aim is to address the challenges experts face in motivating audiences to understand and support public health efforts.

Many of these tools include language (presented in italics) you can use verbatim if you choose to, but you also can tailor the words to your work. This section includes the following:

- A **public health impact formula** that articulates the role of public health in a way that is clear and motivating to non-experts.
- A **unique value proposition** you can use to describe the value delivered by public health and set it apart from other fields.
- A **narrative structure** that organizes key ideas about public health. This framework can be tailored to your work and used to start conversations and generate interest.

- A **one-minute message** and **winning words** to draw on as you shape the narrative to your work.
- Tips for **cutting through the jargon** and replacing technical jargon with memorable, motivating language.

These tools were developed in partnership with Hattaway Communications, a strategic communications firm. The insights and ideas in this toolkit were developed on the basis of an extensive research process, including:

- **Research review:** This review revealed actionable insights and ideas from previous research on public health communications. It also identified lessons from social psychology and cognitive science that show how to communicate with clarity and motivational power.
- **In-depth interviews with public health messengers:** Interviews with fifteen public health practitioners from a range of large, small, urban, and rural health departments across the country explored their challenges communicating about their work and identified the tools, information, and resources they would need in order to be more effective communicators.
- **Focus groups:** Four focus groups were conducted with active citizens—defined in this case as those who vote regularly, meet a threshold of civic and community engagement, and share information about issues that are important to them. These focus groups were conducted in San Jose, California, and Nashville, Tennessee. Participants were recruited to represent a range of ages, genders, races and ethnicities, education levels, income levels, and political

ideologies. These conversations explored the ideas people associate with public health and tested a range of language and messages to help people understand and support the field.

Public health impact formula

The impact formula below articulates the unique functions of public health that

- Leverage the way people intuitively think about their own health
- Differentiate public health from health care
- Motivate people to support public health efforts in their own communities

These concepts help explain the role of public health in a way that is clear and motivating to non-experts (Figure 4.4).

DIAGNOSE

Public health experts diagnose the health of each community by listening to people who live there—then use data, evidence, and research to offer solutions.

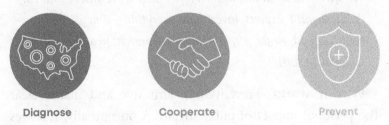

Diagnose   Cooperate   Prevent

Figure 4.4 Diagnose, Cooperate, Prevent.

Why it works: People approach public health by looking for the same things they seek in their own health—customized diagnoses and treatments based on rigorous research and evidence. It is important not to generalize about people's health problems or suggest that public health recommendations are one-size-fits-all.

COOPERATE

To improve the health of the community, different organizations have to work together—schools, businesses, government agencies, and more. Public health brings them together to make decisions and take action.

Why it works: To the degree people associate public health with government, they are nervous that officials are making decisions behind closed doors. Emphasizing cooperation reassures people that public health experts are listening to people in the community. Yet this cooperation must appear action oriented to avoid triggering concerns about bureaucracy.

PREVENT

We often end up in the doctor's office after we're sick or injured. Public health experts investigate everything that affects our health—food, water, air, and more—to prevent health problems before they start.

Why it works: Prevention is intuitive and makes clear the personal impact of public health. Conceptually, it serves as a bridge between personal health and systemic factors. Prevention is also seen as an area where health care under-delivers, and it positions public health as part of the solution to people's frustrations.

Unique value proposition

People are often unclear about the role and value of public health, leading to questions like, "What exactly is public health?" and "How is it different from health care?" The following unique value proposition is a succinct statement that describes the benefits of public health and distinguishes it from other fields. This statement can be used to introduce the topic and answer common questions.

Just as a person makes decisions that affect their health, so does a community. We need clean air and safe neighborhoods, for example. Public health experts listen to the community and look for patterns in what is affecting their health. They use science to diagnose problems, and they bring together everyone who can stop health threats before they start.

Narrative structure

The narrative structure shown below provides a useful method for communicating with maximum motivating power. It includes the pieces that people need in order to understand the "story" of public health. Narratives often flow in the order below—people, goal, problem, solution (Figure 4.5). But you can adjust the order in the way that is most intuitive for your work.

People

Who are the people involved in public health?

Goal

What goals are they working toward?

Problem

What problems stand in the way?

Solution

How will public health solutions benefit individuals and communities?

Figure 4.5 People, Goal, Problem, and Solution.

- **People: Your audience needs to understand the role of public health professionals—and to respect them as people.** Demonstrate that public health professionals are trained experts who draw on science and data—but also emphasize that they listen to, respect, and cooperate with the communities they serve.

- **Goal: People are motivated by aspirations that relate to their own lives.** Members of the public want to avoid their own health problems, so describe how public health helps prevent diseases and injuries that may affect each of us as individuals. Use vivid words and tangible examples, like air, water, and food, that create an image in your audience's mind.

- **Problem: Problems that sound too overwhelming or complex can demotivate audiences, who may feel that an issue is intractable.** Frame the problems that public health addresses as intuitive and solvable. Avoid undermining your audience's sense of personal agency by suggesting that their health is outside their control. Instead, leverage people's frustration with health care— that too much time and money is wasted treating people after there is already a problem.

- **Solution: Your audience will be more inspired and motivated if they can see how your work impacts their lives and communities.** Public health experts bring together everyone who has a role to play in their community's health—schools, businesses, government agencies, and others—to stop health threats before they start.

One-minute message

The statements below express the key ideas—people, goal, problem, solution—from the narrative structure in a message that can be spoken out loud in about a minute. This is one example of how to motivate people to understand and support public health, though you may need to tailor it to your own work.

Public health experts are trained to diagnose the health of a community. They listen to people who know their community best and draw on science and data to recognize patterns and problems. [People]

In the United States, we spend so much time and money on health care, but we're not getting healthier. That's because we wait to treat people until after they're sick or injured. [Problem]

Public health is designed to prevent each of us from getting sick or injured in the first place. Clean air, pure water, safe neighborhoods, and more—it's the mission of public health to make sure our cities, communities, and country have what we need to stay healthy. [Goal]

Public health experts bring together everyone who has a role to play in their community's health—schools, businesses, government agencies, and others—to stop health threats before they start. [Solution]

Winning words

Winning words are the key words and phrases that intuitively connect with people with maximum motivating power and word-of-mouth potential. These winning words help spread your message because they are easy to retain and repeat (Table 4.1).

Cutting through the jargon

One of the biggest challenges in communicating about public health is the use of technical jargon. *Jargon* is a specialized language that people use within a particular professional, cultural, or social group. It has its value: Jargon allows for quick

Table 4.1 Winning Words

Public health experts are trained to diagnose... They draw on science and data.	This language emphasizes that public health professionals are trained experts.
They listen to people who know their community.	Emphasizing that public health experts listen to the community helps alleviate concerns about officials making decisions behind closed doors.
... recognize patterns and problems.	"Patterns" is familiar language that connects the dots between individual health and public health.
We spend so much time and money on health care. We wait to treat people until after they're sick.	Leverage people's frustration with health care–and its lack of prevention–to set up a compelling contrast with public health.
Clean air, pure water, safe neighborhoods...	Vivid examples help people see the role of public health in their lives. Juxtaposing two intuitive examples with a surprising one can help open people's eyes.
Bring together everyone who has a role to play. Stop health threats before they start.	Direct, action-oriented language addresses people's concerns that collaboration can lead to inefficiency.

communication of complex ideas among those who speak the language. But, too often, messengers forget to translate jargon when they're talking to non-experts. When this happens, jargon no longer enables efficient communication—it prevents it.

Fluency theory states that the more easily people understand information, the more likely they are to trust it. The converse is also true: Complexity reduces our ability to think and makes us less likely to understand and believe the information in front of us. When people hear an unfamiliar word, their brain scans verbal memory for clues to its meaning. As their attention turns to this, they literally do not hear what is being said next—and can miss the whole point. For example:

Difficult to process: *Effective care for a mother and her baby at this time also reduces maternal mortality and intrapartum stillbirths, resulting in a triple return on investment.*

Fluent to process: *Effective care for a mother and her baby at this time also saves mothers' lives, keeps babies alive during birth, and saves three times as much money as it costs.*

Collaboration tools: Public health narratives to break down silos

The following section is adapted from "Public Health Narratives to Break Down Silos: A Communication Toolkit to Foster Collaboration," July 2020. Available at www.phrases.org.

The tools in this section can help you build bridges by articulating shared goals, the problems that stand in the way of reaching them, and the solutions that come from partnering with public health professionals.

A growing challenge in public health communications is motivating sector-specific audiences to see the value of collaboration. To successfully break down silos, leaders in other sectors need to understand what public health professionals do and realize the potential benefits of partnering with them.

To meet that need, these tools include research-based language, guidance, and best practices for communicating with sectors such as education, business, health systems, and housing. These tools consist of two sets of research to offer strategic messaging that can help you communicate more effectively with sector-specific audiences.

- **Frame elements:** Sector-specific research conducted by the FrameWorks Institute identified three frame elements that are particularly effective in explaining public health concepts and motivating other sectors to understand the benefits of collaboration. As stated earlier, frame elements are communication devices that alter the presentation (but not the content) of a message—such as a metaphor that helps clarify a concept, a cultural value or shared principle that signals broad relevance, or a particular tone that the messenger adopts. Every communication involves many different frame elements. This toolkit takes these frame elements—designed specifically to close critical gaps in understanding between public health experts and professionals in other sectors—and puts them into practice.

- **Narrative development:** Each frame element identified in the research was translated into a narrative. A narrative is a simple but powerful framework that helps audiences understand complex topics by identifying the people involved, their goals, the problems that stand in the way, and the potential solutions. Insights from psychology and cognitive science inform the most effective words, phrases, and ideas to capture the motivating power of the frame element in a narrative that will be easy to communicate.

These tools can help you communicate more effectively with sector-specific audiences. Throughout, you will find language that you can use verbatim, but in many cases you will want to tailor the words to your work and to the specific sectors you are communicating with.

- **Frame elements** are particularly effective in explaining important concepts in public health and motivating other sectors to see the benefits of collaboration.
- A **narrative structure** organizes key ideas about public health and can help you take each metaphor and translate it into a message about your work.
- A **one-minute message** brings each metaphor to life, and winning words give each message its motivating power.

Frame elements

As described at the beginning of this chapter, research with sector-specific audiences revealed three frame elements that are particularly effective in explaining public health concepts and motivating other sectors to see the benefits of collaboration.

- **The Value of Investment:** This frames how public health professionals work with other sectors to save money in the short term whenever possible and make wise investments over the long term that support community health, increase efficiency, and reduce unnecessary costs for everyone.
- **Foundation of Community Health:** This is a metaphor for how the health of a community is supported by the work of many different sectors. It can also help professionals in other sectors understand the social determinants of health.
- **GPS Navigation:** This is a metaphor for how the field of public health engages data to support the work of other sectors in innovative and forward-thinking ways. GPS is a powerful tool for visualizing and navigating complex terrain, and public health professionals serve this function as well.

To help you put these frame elements into practice, each is shown in the following pages as part of a one-minute message. These messages include language you can use to bring each narrative to life.

One-minute message: The Value of Investment

A message about financial and other benefits of investing in public health that follows the narrative structure is presented below.

Public health experts know that communities only prosper when they're healthy. Their mission isn't just to protect individuals' health—they're making sure businesses, schools, hospitals, and more are set up for success. [People]

Public health is a smart investment: It means a healthy work-force, students ready to learn, and an entire community that knows you're on their side. [Goal]

Too often, we put off thinking about the community's health until there's a problem—a risky gamble that leaves us spending far more money and time digging ourselves out of a hole. [Problem]

When we work together to protect the health of our community, we're protecting the investments we've made in our customers, students, neighbors, and more. [Solution]

Winning words: The Value of Investment

The winning words presented in Table 4.2 are the words and phrases that intuitively connect with people with maximum motivating power and word-of-mouth potential.

Table 4.2 Winning Words: The Value of Investment

Communities only prosper when they're healthy.	This frames collaboration as empowerment and demonstrates that public health experts understand other sectors' needs.
They're making sure businesses, schools, hospitals, and more are set up for success.	
Public health is a smart investment ... a healthy workforce, students ready to learn ...	Keep it positive and paint a vivid picture of the benefits collaboration can offer. You can tailor the imagery here to different sectors.
A risky gamble ... digging ourselves out of a hole.	This conveys that investing in public health is the responsible choice, and it demonstrates familiarity with the challenges many sectors are facing.
Protecting the investments we've made in our customers, students, neighbors ...	Protecting one's investments leverages "loss aversion"—our psychological tendency to fear losses more than we desire gains.

One-minute message: Foundation of Community Health

The following is a message about the role different sectors play in addressing the social determinants of health.

Businesses, schools, hospitals, and government agencies—these are the pillars of communities that support our way of life. With the help of public health experts, they also have a role to play in keeping us healthy. [People]

To have a solid foundation of health, different pillars of a community have to reinforce each other. Students learn best when they have homes that keep them safe and rested; businesses thrive when their employees and customers are healthy. [Goal]

When we wait to treat individual health issues one at a time, we ignore the structural flaws that keep causing problems. [Problem]

Public health professionals can diagnose the health of our community, but they can't fix it alone. Business leaders, educators, and property owners all have the tools we need to build healthy communities. [Solution]

Winning words: Foundation of Community Health

The winning words presented in Table 4.3 are the words and phrases that intuitively connect with people with maximum motivating power and word-of-mouth potential.

Table 4.3 Winning Words: Foundation of Community Health

The pillars of communities that support our way of life . . .	This language builds positive associations with those you hope to motivate and establishes them as key to the foundation metaphor.
To have a solid foundation of health, different pillars of a community have to reinforce each other.	This frames collaboration as mutually beneficial and suggests we're stronger when we build health proactively.
Students learn best when they have homes that keep them safe and rested; businesses thrive when their employees are healthy.	This demonstrates familiarity with other sectors; use vivid language to help them visualize success.
We ignore the structural flaws that keep causing problems.	This frames social determinants within the context of the foundation metaphor and explains how addressing them is in our long-term interest.
All have tools we need to build healthy communities . . .	This frames collaboration as an empowering partnership.

One-minute message: GPS Navigation

The following is a message using the GPS Navigation metaphor to communicate that data expertise is an aid in protecting public health.

Public health experts are trained to spot patterns in data and translate them into concrete actions that leaders in our community—teachers, property owners, business owners, and more—can take to protect our health. [People]

Data help map the steps organizations can take to find innovative solutions to reach their goals more quickly, all while improving the health of their communities. [Goal]

It's easy to get lost in mountains of data. Numbers can point us in different directions and leave organizations feeling stuck.

[Problem]

Partnering with public health experts can provide organizations with a GPS to pinpoint where they are and find the different paths to reach their goals. [Solution]

Winning words: GPS Navigation

The winning words presented in Table 4.4 are the words and phrases that intuitively connect with people with maximum motivating power and word-of mouth potential.

Storytelling tools: Strategic storytelling for public health messengers

The following section is adapted from "Strategic Storytelling for Public Health Messengers: A Research-Based Toolkit," July 2020. Available at www.phrases.org.

The tools in this section will empower you to confidently tell strategic stories about public health. These stories can raise awareness of public health initiatives among key audiences

Table 4.4 Winning Words: GPS Navigation

Public health experts are trained to spot patterns in data.	Foregrounding the data expertise of public health professionals builds confidence they can cut through complexity.
Actions that leaders in our community—teachers, landlords, business owners, and more—can take to protect our health Innovative solutions to reach their goals faster	Put the leaders of other sectors in the picture to show how public health has transformed to meet twenty-first-century needs. Keep it positive: Frame public health as complementing, not competing with, other sectors' goals.
It's easy to get lost in mountains of data . . . leave organizations feeling stuck.	Demonstrate your familiarity with challenges other sectors face. Where possible, insert specific challenges relevant to your audience.
. . . provide organizations with a GPS.	This metaphor frames collaboration as empowerment, and leaves other sectors in the driver's seat.

and inspire those audiences to take action to help achieve your goals. This section includes a number of tools to help you become a more confident storyteller, including the following:

- **The science of storytelling**, including insights from psychology and cognitive science that explain why storytelling is the most effective way to help non-experts understand and embrace a complex topic
- **Strategic storytelling guidance** to ensure that your stories aren't just inspiring but also motivational for the audiences you need to reach
- **Storytelling insights for sector-specific audiences**, offering tailored insights for adapting stories to leaders in housing, education, health systems, business, and other sectors
- **The Public Health Story Map** to help you put pen to paper and begin crafting compelling stories about your work
- **Common storytelling challenges** to help you navigate questions that are likely to arise as you start telling stories about your work

The tools synthesize several bodies of research to offer practical lessons for public health storytelling, including the following:

- **Insights from psychology and cognitive science:** These lessons explain how our brains process information through stories.
- **In-depth interviews with public health messengers:** The FrameWorks Institute conducted interviews with fifteen

public health practitioners from a range of large, small, urban, and rural health departments across the country. These interviews explored their challenges, telling stories about their work, and identified the tools, information, and resources they would need to be more effective storytellers.

- **Focus groups:** Hattaway Communications conducted four focus groups in San Jose, California, and Nashville, Tennessee, with active citizens—defined in this case as those who vote regularly, meet a threshold of civic and community engagement, and share information about issues that are important to them. Participants were recruited to represent a range of demographics. These conversations explored the ideas that people associate with public health and the tangible examples and stories that encourage them to support the field.

- **Research with other sectors:** Research from peer discourse sessions and one-on-one interviews with leaders in business, health care, education, and the housing sector was conducted as part of a Strategic Frame Analysis® by the FrameWorks Institute. Strategic Frame Analysis® is an approach that has been shown to increase understanding of, and engagement in, conversations about public health.

The science of storytelling

Storytelling has always been one of humanity's primary forms of communication. Stories help us make sense of the world, teach us important skills, and inform our sense of right and wrong. Processing information through stories holds several evolutionary advantages. Stories help us

- **Understand cause-and-effect relationships.** Stories are shortcuts that help our brains understand why "this causes that." Understanding cause-and-effect relationships focuses our minds on the people affected by a problem, what caused it, and the people who can change it. This is important in a field like public health—where individuals can seem invisible within a complex system.
- **See patterns in important information.** Our brains strive to recognize patterns that help us make sense of complex information. The desire to identify patterns is why we stay engaged in compelling stories—our brains want to know what's going to happen next. Just as important, identifying patterns in what affects our health can help people understand the need for a public health approach.
- **Empathize with people.** There's a reason we find ourselves crying during sad movies and on edge during horror films. Our brains have "mirror neurons" that mimic the emotions of people we observe. Because of this, stories give us the power to help our audience empathize with others, including those who would benefit from public health programs and policies.
- **Pay attention.** Stories engage a much larger part of our brain than other information. Different parts of our brain are responsible for processing sights, sounds, vivid imagery, emotions, and so on. When we tell a story that stimulates these senses, our brains fire on more cylinders—which means we're more likely to pay attention and remember what we're hearing.

These insights help explain why storytelling is one of the most effective forms of communication and is especially well suited for communications about public health. In the following pages, we'll share practical steps for crafting strategic stories about your work.

Strategic storytelling guidance

To help achieve your goals, the stories you tell need to be strategic. A strategic story is not merely interesting or inspirational—it is designed to motivate a specific audience. Crafting strategic stories starts with a clear understanding of your audience and your purpose. You can get started by answering a few basic questions:

- **What is your shared goal for collaboration?** Clearly articulate a specific goal that you are working together toward. Be vivid, and give the audience a picture of how their community or world will be safer, healthier, and more prosperous if your work is successful. In a story, you can help your audience envision your goal by describing your protagonist's aspirations. ("She hopes to live in a community where . . .")
- **Who can help you achieve that goal?** Your audience should walk away understanding their role in helping you reach an outcome. Keep it positive by focusing on what your audience can add. Include characters like them in your story so they can empathize with the people their actions will benefit.

- **What do you want your audience to know, feel, and do?**
  Stories can affect an audience in three ways: increase their awareness, change their attitude, or inspire them to action. Plan how you want to influence your audience—what you want them to know, feel, or do after hearing your story—so that you can adjust the story accordingly.

  - **Know:** What do you hope your story will make them more aware of?
  - **Feel:** What emotions do you hope your story will provoke?
  - **Do:** What actions should your story motivate them to take?

Storytelling insights for sector-specific audiences

The Public Health Story Map can be used to tell stories to any audience, including the general public. However, research identified specific insights that can inform stories aimed at sector-specific audiences, including housing, business, education, and health systems. Following are descriptions of those insights and how the Public Health Story Map can help you address them.

- **Share vivid success stories that link cross-sector collaborations to the concrete benefits they deliver.** Other sectors may not understand how collaboration would work. The Public Health Story Map will help you share memorable success stories that help audiences visualize how you would work together.

- **Illustrate how the field of public health is transforming to meet twenty-first century needs.** Audiences from other sectors may have an outdated view of public health's role. Stories can help you demonstrate how public health has evolved to protect health in an interconnected world.
- **Leverage allies and public health professionals working in or with other sectors as messengers.** Sector-specific audiences are proud of their expertise and may not see how public health experts can add to it. The Public Health Story Map demonstrates how to bring in allies from other sectors to validate your work.
- **Frame collaboration as empowerment.** Other sectors can be wary of being told what to do. The Public Health Story Map will help you tell stories that demonstrate how collaboration is mutually beneficial.
- **Foreground public health's data expertise.** Sector-specific audiences see the value in concrete data that helps them navigate challenges. The Public Health Story Map identifies how to incorporate data expertise into a story without making it technical or dry.
- **Keep it positive.** Being alarmist can demotivate other sectors from wanting to collaborate. The Public Health Story Map can help you frame challenges as opportunities and share examples of constructive actions that audiences can take.

The Public Health Story Map: How to craft strategic stories

To help tell stories about public health, Hattaway Communications created the Public Health Story Map (Figure 4.6).

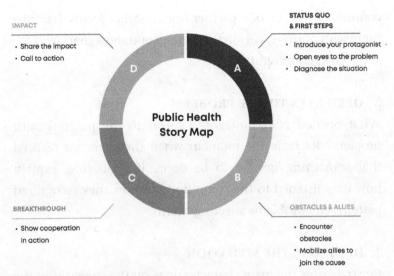

Figure 4.6 Public Health Story Map.

It is adapted from the Hero's Journey, a tried-and-true model used to structure stories that capture people's attention and imagination. It is a "formula" based on research about storytelling across different cultures. Familiarizing yourself with the Public Health Story Map will help you craft stories; it also will help you identify stories by yielding clues about what elements to look for.

The Public Health Story Map helps structure your story around a narrative arc. There are eight steps for mapping a story from beginning to end—some stories will cover all the steps, and some will touch on only a few.

1. INTRODUCE YOUR PROTAGONIST

Begin by describing the main characters of your story. They may be you or another public health official, a local activist or community leader, or a partner from another sector. Describe them with positive, personal attributes and show that they care about their community.

2. OPEN EYES TO THE PROBLEM

What opened your protagonist's eyes to the public health problem? Recreate the moment when the character realized that something needed to be done. If applicable, explain how they listened to the community or how they recognized patterns and problems affecting health.

3. DIAGNOSE THE SITUATION

Illustrate how the main character drew on the strengths of the public health field—data, evidence, and research—to understand what was happening and develop ideas for addressing it.

4. ENCOUNTER OBSTACLES

What challenges did your characters encounter that prevented them from solving this problem on their own? An obstacle should be significant but not overwhelming. Avoid complex jargon that can make the problem seem confusing or unsolvable.

5. MOBILIZE ALLIES TO JOIN THE CAUSE

Describe the community members or organizations that have a role in addressing this problem. If this is a story targeted to a specific sector, make sure to include individuals from those sectors here (if they are not already the main protagonist).

Putting the audience in the story as allies can help potential partners envision how they might get involved.

6. SHOW COOPERATION IN ACTION
Cooperation between sectors is motivating, but it should be action oriented rather than bureaucratic. What actions did everyone take? Describe their can-do attitude and how they cooperated, made decisions, and supported common goals. If relevant, explain how public health leaders helped facilitate this cooperation.

7. SHARE THE IMPACT
Describe how people's lives were changed for the better, being as specific as possible about the tangible benefits for everyone involved. For the public, explain how future health problems were prevented. For sector-specific audiences, explain how they helped achieve their own goals or saw a return on their investment.

8. CALL TO ACTION
Your story has inspired and informed people. Now, what can they do to advance the cause? To create a sense of urgency, describe what will be gained by acting soon and what will be lost by waiting. Tell your audience exactly what they can do, and make it easy for them to act.

Common storytelling challenges
There are three types of stories that public health experts may find especially difficult to craft:

- Stories when there is no impact (yet)
- Stories about systems change
- Stories of lessons learned from failure

Following are recommendations for tackling each of these challenges.

TELLING STORIES WHEN THERE IS NO IMPACT (YET)

What if the story you'd like to tell doesn't end with progress being made? That can be a positive thing. Research shows that stories with a too-happy ending can be demotivating because they make the audience feel as though the work is already done. If your story lacks signs of change, focus instead on articulating your vision and creating a sense of urgency to help realize it.

Articulate your vision

- **Be aspirational.** As you reach the end of your story, transition to the future tense and focus on your vision for change, or refer to other instances in which similar work has been successful. Describe the healthier world the protagonist is trying to shape and how life for them—and even your audience—will be better if their efforts are successful.
- **Be vivid.** Psychological research shows that people are more motivated to work toward goals they can see in their mind's eye. When describing your aspirational vision, use vivid words that describe people, places, or things—and avoid abstract language or health jargon that people can't visualize.

Create a sense of urgency

- Even if you haven't achieved your ultimate goal, talk about people doing something to get there and describe the positive emotions that correspond with getting involved. Is there a sense of unity, momentum, or personal fulfillment? Articulating these emotional benefits can motivate people to help you reach the finish line.

TELLING STORIES ABOUT SYSTEMS CHANGE

Public health professionals often address systemic health inequalities and problems that arise within complex, bureaucratic systems. Given that, you may wonder whether you can craft a compelling story about systems change. Good stories are about interesting characters—and systems are about rules, policies, and norms. But the divide between the two is not as wide as you may think. Systems, after all, are the results of actions by individuals over time. Those systems affect individuals—and they can be changed by individuals. To translate systems change into compelling stories, you simply have to pinpoint the right characters.

- **Focus on a protagonist within the system.** A common misconception is that stories need to focus exclusively on the people who benefit from a cause. While that is an effective approach, you can also craft a compelling story about people who are embedded in a system or who have the power to create change. Public health professionals can be inspiring protagonists, as they have deep knowledge of the systems that affect health and are well positioned to effect change.

- **Avoid overwhelming your audience with complexity.**
Public health professionals have an understandable desire
to communicate the complexity of systems change to their
audiences—but this can backfire. People tend to avoid
problems that seem overwhelming because they feel pow-
erless to solve them. Breaking down complex systems into
specific, solvable problems can help motivate your audience to take action and make for a more compelling story.

TELLING STORIES ABOUT LESSONS LEARNED FROM FAILURE

Stories about lessons learned from failure don't have to
be demotivating. They can be the vehicle for sharing key
takeaways and can speak to the way you approach problems.
Other public health experts may be able to refine their work
based on your insights, and external audiences will see that
you are committed to refining your approach. Effective stories
about failure should describe your goal, what went wrong, and
what you plan to do differently.

- **Talk about what the goal was and why it was a worthy
effort.** Even though you failed to achieve your goal, it's
important to let your audience know what that goal was
and why it is still worth pursuing. This will keep listeners
focused on what can be achieved if you succeed and why
they should continue to support the effort.
- **Be specific about what went wrong and when you
realized it.** Demonstrating that you understand exactly what went wrong shows that you learned from the

experience and builds confidence that the next effort will be more successful. One way to do this effectively in a story is to recreate the moment when you or your protagonist realized what went wrong. Helping your audiences understand the emotions of that moment will create empathy and get them to care more about your eventual success.

- **Discuss what worked.** Even though you didn't achieve your ultimate goal, discussing what did work will build confidence in elements of your approach and motivate others to replicate them. If you built a lasting partnership, talk about what worked for both sides. Showing how close you came to success creates a sense of urgency to get the job done and makes your goal seem within reach.

- **Be aspirational and discuss what you're going to do next.** Demonstrate that you're better positioned to succeed in the future because of what you've learned. What do you know now that you can immediately apply to your next effort? Include an aspirational vision of what you can accomplish with these newfound lessons.

More resources

Visit www.phrases.org for additional communications resources, including a Quick Start Guide, the "Map the Gaps" report, a Strategic Framing Brief, and the following tools:

- **When You Say . . . They Think**
  When communicating with sectors outside of public health, often what we say comes across in a very different way than anticipated. This tool shows commonly used

phrases from public health, explains what another sector might be thinking in reaction, and provides framing tips and guidance for reframing our communications.

- **Answers to Tough Questions**
PHRASES crowdsourced tough questions about public health that practitioners are often confronted with, such as "What is public health?" and "How is public health different from health care?" This tool shows a standard or typical answer to the question, plus a reframed answer.

- **Sample Emails**
Outreach emails are often an important early communication between public health professionals and other sectors. This tool has before-and-after versions of a sample introductory communication to initiate a cross-sector partnership.

- **Sample Documents**
This tool offers examples of strategic plans, memoranda of understanding, governance structures, and logic models for public health professionals to adapt in their collaboration work.

- **Resource Library**
The PHRASES library includes resources on framing and collaboration, including websites, articles, blog posts, fact sheets, reports, and toolkits.

Part III
Bringing Public Health to Life

5

How to Tell Impactful Stories

SOLEDAD O'BRIEN AND ROSE ARCE

EARLY IN 2020, OUR TEAM WAS in Seattle filming a documentary on homelessness. After production started, we realized that another public health crisis was emerging: Seattle had become ground zero for COVID-19 in the United States. Our plans quickly changed. What began as a story about homelessness expanded to show the compounding burdens of life during a pandemic.

"Outbreak: The First Response," produced with support from the de Beaumont Foundation, is an account of the first days of the COVID-19 outbreak in the Seattle area. The documentary follows two residents and their families who were especially vulnerable to the pandemic: Stevie Habedank, who was living out of a car with her boyfriend and daughter, and Katherine Kempf, whose father, living in a long-term care facility, had tested positive for COVID-19. Viewers watch the hardships that Stevie and Katherine each face in protecting their families, and

Soledad O'Brien and Rose Arce, *How to Tell Impactful Stories* In: *Talking Health*. Edited by: Mark R. Miller, Brian C. Castrucci, Rachel Locke, Julia Haskins, and Grace A. Castillo, Oxford University Press.
© de Beaumont Foundation 2022. DOI: 10.1093/oso/9780197528464.003.0006

they get a glimpse of public health on the ground, as officials such as Patty Hayes, health director for Seattle-King County, manage complicated response efforts. "Outbreak" is more than a narrative of the pandemic; it is also a story of public health and the lives it touches.

Stories are powerful. They can shift our thinking and help us see issues from new perspectives. They can entertain us or shake us to our core. Now that all eyes are on public health in the wake of the pandemic, it is a critical moment for telling stories about the work being done to support the health and well-being of communities. With the principles of good storytelling, you can explain, celebrate, and advocate for public health. Here's how to tell impactful stories as a public health practitioner.

Talk like a real person

Every industry has its jargon, which is useful under the right circumstances. If you want to refer to "the social determinants of health" at a professional conference, go for it. But when you're talking to people who don't have a background in public health, you need to explain concepts in ways they'll understand. Instead of "social determinants of health," use a straightforward description like "conditions that affect our health and well-being, including the environment and access to housing and education."

Imagine you're talking to a friend or family member. Your grandmother doesn't need the textbook definition of public health practice. She'll be more inclined to listen if you speak to her naturally. So, tell her about how you help people lead healthier, longer lives and what that work entails.

When you work in a world of high-level science, it's easy to lose touch with people outside of your sphere. Don't try to impress people with your knowledge or by insulting their intelligence. The best storytellers aren't the ones who have the most sophisticated vocabularies, but the ones who communicate information clearly and simply.

Make relevant connections

Talking about public health is especially hard if you go into a conversation cold. When you can help people make meaningful, relevant connections to the field in their own lives, you're more likely to win hearts and minds.

Maybe the person you're talking to doesn't know much about epidemiology but they understand the severity of an infectious disease outbreak. Explain that epidemiologists track the spread of disease and collaborate with other public health experts to protect their communities. Their investigative efforts prevented countless deaths and infections throughout the COVID-19 pandemic, as well as during other outbreaks that didn't make the headlines.

Take that example a step further and discuss the importance of investing in public health. How much better prepared for the pandemic could we have been had epidemiologists been equipped to do their jobs more effectively? Could more lives have been saved if funding for public health was on par with that for the military?

Of course, it's not all about crises. Elevate the work of non-emergency roles in public health, like sanitarians, who assess environmental health and safety in schools and factories. Your audience will appreciate your story more if you explain the impact that their sanitarian has made on their community, like ensuring that food safety regulations are in place at their favorite local restaurant. They have a sanitarian to thank for a clean, healthy dining experience that possibly kept them from becoming ill.

Start small

Public health by definition deals with populations. The problem is that we struggle to wrap our minds around big numbers and large groups of people—in other words, public health stories. Eyes will glaze over if you prepare your audience for an account of 6,000 people, no matter how captivating the tale may be. Creating an emotional connection on that scale doesn't work. The trick for public health professionals is to tell the story of one person who is representative of many.

The most compelling narratives in journalism often begin with someone who exemplifies a larger conflict or trend. This person serves as the hook, drawing in the reader, listener, or viewer as you move into big-picture themes. Opening a story through the eyes of a person seeking shelter in the wake of a hurricane is more gripping than stating that thousands of people were forced to evacuate their homes. Instead of describing the scene at a relief center filled with people waiting for donations, focus on one person anxiously awaiting news about her family.

Once you've established that single person's story, you can delve further into the systems that have succeeded or failed in supporting populations, which go far beyond clinical interventions. Public health may be the story of many, but it is more powerfully communicated through the individual.

Make data come to life

Data and storytelling go hand in hand. When woven into narratives with moving anecdotes, data can take stories to new heights.

Public health professionals often hesitate to go outside the data set when telling a story. The standard who, what, when, where, and why are all there, but the story falls flat without a closer look at the people behind the statistics. To add color, seek out real stories from people at the center of events in public health. If the research you're communicating is about maternal and child health, find the mother who will speak to you about the barriers she has encountered getting formula for her baby or securing affordable child care.

Another way to make data engaging is through equations that show how something may or may not have occurred as a result of public health interventions. For instance, you can point to how a community with a certain number of vaccinations had lower rates of flu than a community that failed to bolster vaccinations. This framing gives proof of life to public health efforts, showing the benefits of investing in the field or the devastating effects of underfunding.

Find the value in all stories

Public health deals with population-wide challenges that aren't always rosy. That doesn't mean you should scrap the story you want to tell because it's not uplifting enough. All that matters is that your story is real.

Stories tend to be framed within a positive–negative binary that says a kid's lemonade stand is good and a tornado is bad. But this reductive stance overlooks the nuances that make stories worth telling. A better approach is to consider what aspects are most intriguing, regardless of the gravity of the subject.

Take the example of a story about climate change. Who are the people rallying their local policymakers? Is there a scientist helping non-experts make sense of the data? What are community members doing to put pressure on the biggest polluters? Most of all, how is public health making a difference?

Looking at what is being done to address a social problem—not dwelling solely on the issue itself—is the goal of solutions journalism. When you tell stories about public health, focus on the solutions that practitioners and allies are implementing in communities. Plenty of stories have emerged from adversities, and there always are examples of resilience, passion, and hope in the worst circumstances.

Tell your story—again and again

Public health professionals begin at a disadvantage when telling stories because their field isn't well understood. Be prepared to repeat your stories, as obvious as they may seem to you. Chances are that your audience will be surprised to learn about the scale and scope of the public health workforce.

When an outbreak of hepatitis A was declared in Washington State in 2019, many residents weren't even aware that a crisis had occurred. The word didn't get out that public health practitioners were there from the start, working to prevent further spread and protect the most vulnerable community members, especially homeless populations. Every time an event like this happens, public health needs to be vocal about the role of practitioners and the impact they've made on communities. Otherwise, that narrative disappears.

We saw this happen during the COVID-19 pandemic, when heart-wrenching stories of nurses and doctors serving on the frontlines of the response made most of the headlines. Health care became the dominant narrative, even though its practitioners were treating people who were sick, which was a more limited role than that of public health professionals, who were managing the community-wide response. You need to keep telling your story to give it the respect and attention it deserves in a crowded media market.

Put yourself out there

In the twenty-four-hour cable news cycle, politicians with no scientific expertise can weigh in on climate change and infectious disease just because they've maneuvered their way into a time slot. Whenever possible, public health professionals should be the ones on camera, not the talking heads.

You need to push to include yourself and your colleagues in conversations about public health. Find the people in your organization who have both the expertise and the personality to give a compelling interview when a news outlet calls. Then, make introductions with reporters in your community who cover topics across the spectrum of public health. Get comfortable pestering network and local TV executives to make sure that the right person is tapped to be the voice of issues related to public health when opportunities arise.

If traditional media isn't an option, turn to the social media platforms at your disposal. Host a Twitter chat or answer questions from community members on an Instagram or Facebook livestream.

Governmental public health employees who are restricted in speaking to the media can still raise the profile of their field by communicating through elected officials and other high-profile figures. Even if you aren't the one being quoted, you can ensure that people in the spotlight are sharing consistent, science-based public health messaging with the people they serve.

Tell stories for the greater good

Storytelling is a force for change in public health. When you talk about what it means to work in public health, you're taking steps toward building support and awareness, both of which the field desperately needs.

The more you tell the stories of public health, the more people will begin to think differently about what matters most when it comes to their well-being and longevity. They will begin to realize that health is not just about what happens within the four walls of a hospital; in fact, policies, systems, and environments actually have more influence on their health.

There is no shortage of incredible stories about public health, and you likely have many of your own from personal experience. They need to be communicated in a way that resonates with people outside the field.

Reflect on what you have seen, heard, or felt as a public health professional and how that can translate into a moving story. What struck a chord that you want other people to know? As you formulate your stories, consider how they might inspire action on behalf of public health. You could be the spark that brings more attention to your local health department or leads to sweeping policy changes. It all begins with a story.

This is your opportunity to shift the conversation about public health, one that leaves a lasting impact. You have the knowledge, expertise, and experience to tell stories that will get people to care about public health well into the future. Go out and make sure the world hears them.

6

Think Like a Marketer: Find Your Hook, Make It Beautiful, and Humanize the Numbers

SARAH MARTIN, WITH CONTRIBUTIONS BY ANNA DUIN

EVERY DAY, THE FORCES THAT SEEK to keep people unhealthy pour billions of dollars into marketing and storytelling. Armed with teams of psychologists, economists, and creators, companies use communication to create emotional connections to their brands. Public health as a field has not kept up. The further we fall behind, the more likely it is that our framework for health equity will fail and these disparities will persist.

When public health leaders are ignored, people die

If leaders in public health want to sway audiences outside their own field, they have to play the game. To bring public health to life, do what any good salesperson would do: find your hook,

Sarah Martin, with contributions by Anna Duin, *Think Like a Marketer* In: *Talking Health*. Edited by: Mark R. Miller, Brian C. Castrucci, Rachel Locke, Julia Haskins, and Grace A. Castillo, Oxford University Press. © de Beaumont Foundation 2022. DOI: 10.1093/oso/9780197528464.003.0007 make it beautiful, and humanize the numbers. This chapter covers these three concepts, focusing on the words, images, and data that will best elevate the public health brand.

Find your hook: Words matter

> Many years later, as he faced the firing squad, Colonel Aureliano Buendía was to remember that distant afternoon when his father took him to discover ice.
>
> —Opening line of *One Hundred Years of Solitude*, by Gabriel García Márquez (1967)

The first words of a good book capture your imagination and make you want to read more. Experienced authors obsess over this make-or-break first impression, and you should, too. If you think you're spending too much time focusing on your first words, you're doing something right.

Examples of compelling leading statements

The following leading statements are used by state or local health department partners of mySidewalk. They are bold and easy to understand. Each gives you a sense of *why* the department does what it is doing. At mySidewalk, we call these top-level statements "power pitches," and they represent the opportunity to quickly persuade an audience to keep reading.

- "Behavioral health is real health" —Community Health Improvement Plan dashboard for Clay County, Florida
- "We need stability, not stress, from our homes" —dashboard generator for Blue Shield of California

- "The American Dream is not a reality for all."—Community Health Assessment dashboard for Kansas City, Missouri
- "Prevention is the fiscally responsible policy choice." —Community Health Improvement Plan dashboard for Maricopa County, Arizona
- "You can't keep a job if you can't get to it." —Community Health Improvement Plan dashboard for Wyandotte County, Kansas

Craft your power pitch

Simple reflection questions can help craft your power pitch. Think of it as a tree: Shared values are the roots, the opportunity is the trunk, and the resolution is the branches.

The roots: Shared values and your *why*

- What is something that most people, no matter their politics, would agree on?
  - Example: *Everyone deserves to live a long, healthy life.*
- What should everyone in your community have that you're trying to deliver?
  - Example: *Everyone deserves to live in a safe neighborhood.*

The trunk: Your central opportunity statement (also known as the "problem statement")

- Why isn't your vision a reality?
  - Example: *X% of kids go to sleep almost every night hearing gunshots.*
  - Example: *We know that X% of moms in Anytown will lose their baby before their first birthday.*

The branches: Multiple ways for your work to address the opportunity

- What is the natural connection between your work and the needs of the community? (This is the place to spell out what support you need.)
  - Example: *This is why the Anytown Health Department wants your input on the new Child Health Improvement Plan.*

Pro tip: Keep your language straightforward. Research shows that if your message is above the seventh-grade level, comprehension drops significantly.

Flip the script

Many public health practitioners feel comfortable presenting the facts but don't know how to make them compelling. Very few public sector agencies do message testing as consistently or frequently as the private sector, and so the story of the "product" they are selling is less developed than for an ordinary consumer good. Training programs that are not housed in a business or management school devote very little time to teaching and explaining social marketing.

In a recent webinar by mySidewalk, we asked attendees (from both the public and private health sectors): "If Public Health were a person, what type of person would they be?"

The answers from many private-sector attendees were unsurprising:

Public health is like my teacher, nagging me not to vape.

Public health reminds me of that strait-laced friend we all had—
the one always telling me everything fun we're doing is bad.

Many people see the larger field of public health as taking things *away* from them. But public safety professionals, such as firefighters, are seen as heroes. As one of mySidewalk's customers put it: "Public health dares to go where no one else will. It presses on when everyone else has given up." As a public health professional, you save lives and make communities better, and that's the brand public health should have.

Communicating about COVID-19 is an example of an opportunity to retell a story for maximum influence. It's easy to focus your health message on the need for social distancing, the importance of masks, and changing infection rates. Detractors of public health policy have framed those mandates as "taking things away"—connection, jobs, freedom. If you don't intentionally tell your own story, someone else will tell it for you—and government overreach is a compelling story.

Flipping the script from a narrative of deprivation to a story of gains helps people in your community widen their perspective. It casts public health in a more essential role.

The truest story is that public health leaders have spent decades advocating for initiatives that don't take things away from people but instead *add* to their lives. You didn't revoke a group's right to smoke indoors—you gave clean air to millions. You didn't force unnecessary regulations on restaurant owners—you protected every man, woman, person, and child in your city from potentially fatal food poisoning. You provide safety, security, and peace of mind.

Disrupt mental shortcuts with better framing

The brain often resorts to stereotypes. As we process information, our minds automatically make subconscious connections between data points. This is called a *heuristic*, or a mental shortcut. Humans are conditioned to be biased, in that they attribute outcomes to the characteristics of the people involved. Your story may be perpetuating these biases.

Think of the commonly repeated fact that "people of color are more likely to get sick from COVID-19." The underlying message is that there is something about these people that makes them get sicker than others. It creates an "us" and "them" mentality that can quickly turn antagonistic. Society has conditioned us to blame people for what happens to them, based on characteristics they can't change.

The good news is you can disrupt habits and heuristics by using better words and images that connect individual outcomes to shared responsibility (see Figure 6.1).

Shifting the frame	OUR COMMUNITY
VULNERABLE POPULATIONS	A virus = biological. Who gets it, lives, and dies = biological + social + economical + political.
It's people who are old, vulnerable, and already sick who are most likely to get Covid-19.	If we are going to emerge stronger, knowledge is power. Explore our CHA with our interactive dashboard.

Figure 6.1 Shifting the Frame to Connect Individual Outcomes With Shared Responsibility. Community Health Assessment.

Make it beautiful: All about aesthetics

Most official documents go unread. We hear public health professionals say that they have lots of data but they don't know how to make it interesting. As one epidemiologist in Southern California put it, "I know data, but I don't know pretty."

Not enough "pretty" is a problem. Your audience's brains process images 60,000 times faster than text, and 90 percent of the information processed by the brain is visual. Research also shows that presentations that include visual aids such as photos, charts, maps, or infographics are 43 percent more persuasive.

According to research by the Kirwan Institute, "the visual representation of social problems within the community elicited different, stronger reactions than just the presentation of raw numbers." The research found that "opportunity mapping" helped state officials "see the severity of the problem."

Place-based data stories and images are especially engaging. Officials in Kansas City, Missouri, for example, saw an increase in resident engagement with their Community Health Improvement Plan when they transitioned from a static report to an interactive map showing life expectancy rates. The original document was downloaded thirty-seven times in the course of the year, while the online life expectancy map received 340 unique engagements in the first six weeks of publication.

Guiding principles for beautiful data

As with fashion, simple data are sophisticated. Clean, straightforward data are powerful. Avoid loud colors and busy graphics—they can distract from the story you're trying to tell.

User experience (UX) is critical. Details such as a reading level above seventh grade and dense charts can quickly alienate people. Your story should be easy to understand, accessible to persons with disabilities, and mobile-friendly. If you don't have a gift for user experience (UX) design, recruit someone who does. Consider this passage from a community health assessment at two different grade levels:

Upper-level college:

We know that education alone isn't enough to reduce chronic disease—but we also know we can't achieve health equity without it. Making sure that everyone has access to the latest information and feels empowered to understand the disease is an essential public health service that the health department is ready to provide.

Seventh-grade level:

Sometimes it's hard to make healthy choices, even when you know it's the right thing to do. A healthier city is about more than education. A healthier Anytown is full of excited, connected people who want to make good choices. The health department is responsible for making sure residents have the ability and the desire to do so.

Use a variety of visuals, and make sure the takeaway is obvious. Leverage maps, charts, and pictures. If a quick pass of your story shows that most of the visuals are bar charts, consider including some other type of visual, like a photo, so that redundancy doesn't bore the reader. Ensure that your chart titles summarize the main takeaway from the visuals, for those who might struggle to interpret the analysis.

Best-dressed public documents

By tracking average page views and average read time, our partners have learned a lot about what works and what doesn't for public health storytelling. One lesson is abundantly clear: titles and style matter.

Let's start with titles. Which would you rather pick up and skim: "City of Townsville Budget 2020" or "Prosperity for All: The Townsville Blueprint for Success"? The first sounds like a paperweight and the other sounds like a page-turner.

Think of the last government or nonprofit report, budget, or publication you've seen. It probably looked something like what appears in Figure 6.2.

The cover of that document doesn't imply a riveting read. We think something like the cover shown in Figure 6.3 is much more beautiful.

Figure 6.4 shows another example that has it all: people, industry, some nature, and some skyline. Plus, the term "century agenda" gives us goosebumps.

A little creativity, free photos from sites like Unsplash, and simple, no-cost design tools like Canva can make a big difference. Ensure that your images don't deepen implicit biases and heuristics; they shouldn't connect things like race and poverty or imply that only a certain perceived gender can do a particular job. Make sure you know your audience's values and motivations, and align your images accordingly.

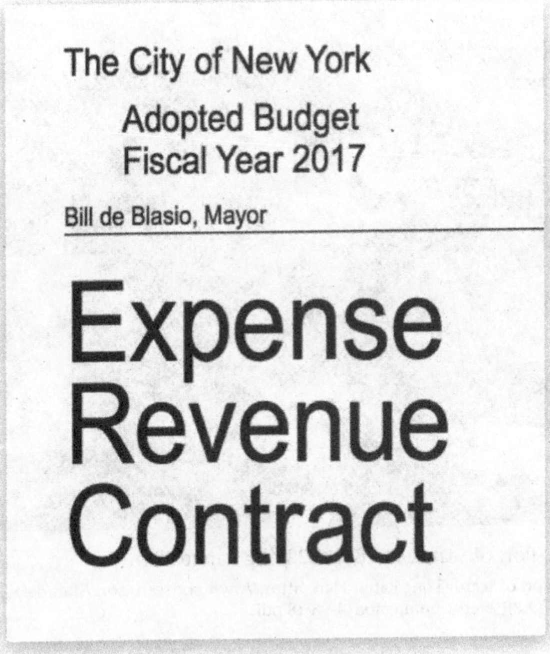

The City of New York

Adopted Budget
Fiscal Year 2017

Bill de Blasio, Mayor

Expense
Revenue
Contract

Figure 6.2 New York City Expense Revenue Contract.

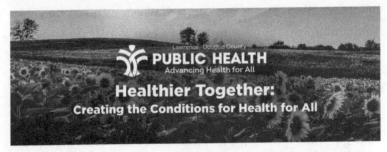

Figure 6.3 Healthier Together: Creating the Conditions of Health for All.
Image from Lawrence Douglas County dashboard. https://dashboards.mysidewalk.com/health
iertogether.

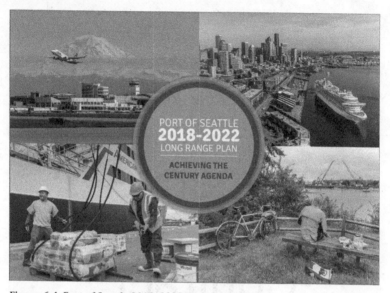

Figure 6.4 Port of Seattle 2018–2022 Long Range Plan.
Image from Port of Seattle Long Range Plan. https://www.portseattle.org/sites/default/files/2018-05/POS_2017_LRP_Web_Commission_4-26-18.pdf.

Not all official documents can be *New York Times* bestsellers, but they still can drive engagement; they can matter to your audience. Start by asking yourself, "Does this sound like something I would want to read? Does it look interesting?" If you'd want to read it, chances are your community members will, too.

Prove it to them: Humanize your data

Many people see the phrase "humanize the data" and think this means the marriage of narrative storytelling and data visualization. While this is an important aspect, we like to think of that phrase more holistically. At mySidewalk, we spend a lot of time examining how the data can come alive for the consumer in a way that reveals the human story within.

One of the first questions to ask about your health data is, "What am I trying to convey and why am I choosing to show the data this way?" Is it intentional, or is it just a habit?

The choice of your geographic unit of analysis is something you likely do reflexively. But you have to treat this choice with mindfulness of the reader's humanity. Choose geographies that mean something to them, even if it is harder for you. If your readers don't know their census tract number, will they see themselves in your data? Census tracts may provide more granularity for researchers (Figure 6.5), but city council districts or neighborhoods will capture attention faster (Figure 6.6).

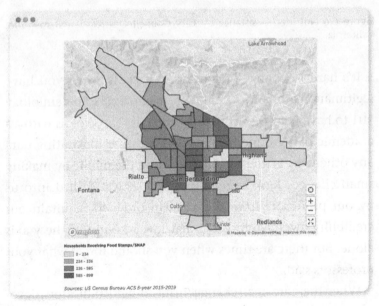

Figure 6.5 Nutrition Assistance by Census Tract, San Bernardino, California.

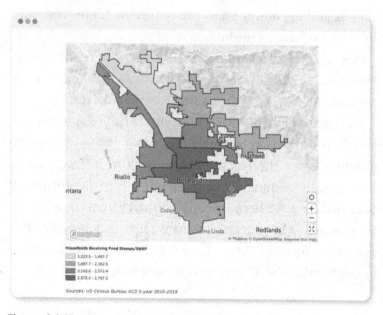

Figure 6.6 Nutrition Assistance by City Council District, San Bernardino, California.

It's hard to change your ways, especially when you have legitimate reasons for them. For example, it's Epidemiology 101 to have graphs start with a zero axis. Those of us with an academic background may have heard that illustrating data any other way is unethical. Misleading the public by making small changes look large is immoral. It was drilled into us by our professors from day one: In order to maintain our credibility, we have to leave that lower bound of the y-axis alone. But there are times when you should forget what your professors said.

When there are small changes in meaningful indicators, devotion to the textbooks can ignore human lives. A one-percentage point change in a condition or disease, for example, can be hundreds or thousands of people, depending on the population. A one-percentage-point change in rural Arizona will not take the same human toll as it will in Los Angeles. But a dogmatic devotion to a zero axis in Los Angeles can invalidate the lives and deaths of those people. Their stories matter, too.

What's a public health leader to do? Show it both ways. Consider the following real data on the number of adults in Kansas City, Missouri, with self-rated poor mental health. Over the course of three years, the prevalence of poor mental health increased by 1.5 percentage points. The gravity of that shift for the three thousand people newly experiencing poor mental health should be highlighted. At the same time, we need to recognize the increase proportionate to overall prevalence in the community. Figures 6.7 and 6.8 show the same data with two different axis choices.

Ultimately, data are most effective when you view it from multiple angles and consider what will best connect your message to your audience with truth and clarity.

Here are some other tips for displaying data in a compelling story:

- Break down data in multiple formats, such as census, zip code, and political district.
- Don't use only national averages; localize baseline metrics to your community.
- Think about using an asset-based approach instead of a vulnerability approach. Instead of focusing on data that show risk, use the inverse of those measures to show resilience.

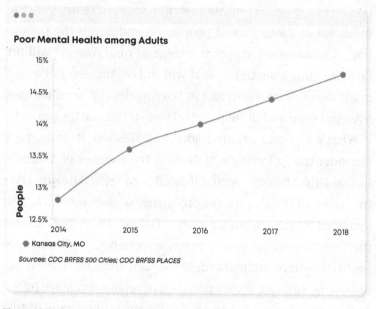

Poor Mental Health among Adults

Figure 6.7 Poor Mental Health among Adults.

A one-percentage-point change in Kansas City, Missouri, can account for more than three thousand additional individuals with poor mental health.

The last word (for now)

Attention to detail adds up. Small tweaks make a big difference in how much engagement your story will get. If your story is rooted in equity, you've already accomplished the most important part. We emphasize concepts like messaging, design, and humanization because our primary goal is to ensure that public health is valued by the community and adequately supported by those in power.

Small steps—like testing your messages with a diverse audience, checking your narrative reading level and design accessibility, and using free tools to make your work more visually

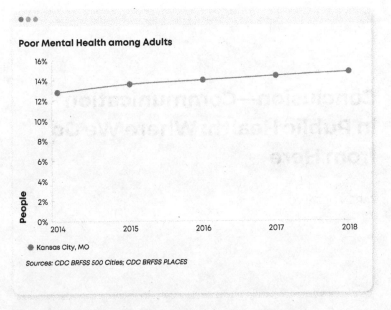

Figure 6.8 Poor Mental Health among Adults.
This graph, with the 'people' axis beginning at 0 percent, at does not illustrate the point as effectively.

appealing—will yield high returns on engagement and positive public opinion. Make a commitment today in your organization to take one of these actions. By telling better stories and leveraging what works, you will capture not only the attention of your audience but also the respect needed to make lasting improvements to community health.

Conclusion—Communication in Public Health: Where We Go from Here

KAREN DESALVO

WHEN I ARRIVED AT THE NEW ORLEANS Health Department as health commissioner, the agency was undergoing an effort to explain its components and how they worked together to support community health. Residents didn't understand the role of the department, and it wasn't clear to them how divisions like environmental health or emergency preparedness fit into a larger framework for protecting health across all stages of life.

Part of my job was to connect the dots in a way that would resonate with the people we served. Communicating the role of the health department was the first step in getting stakeholders and community members to respect, recognize, and invest in us over the long term. But this seemingly straightforward task was easier said than done. How do you get people to care about

Karen DeSalvo, *Conclusion—Communication in Public Health* In: *Talking Health*. Edited by: Mark R. Miller, Brian C. Castrucci, Rachel Locke, Julia Haskins, and Grace A. Castillo, Oxford University Press.
© de Beaumont Foundation 2022. DOI: 10.1093/oso/9780197528464.003.0008

what you do when your field has long struggled to articulate its worth and influence?

As we have seen time and again, communication can be challenging—but it is key to successful public health practice. One of the clearest examples of the power of communication came during the COVID-19 pandemic. Throughout the crisis, public health professionals flexed their communication skills in a range of planning and response initiatives. Practitioners got up to speed on strategies to build trust with communities and help them comply with evidence-based guidance. They employed culturally competent language to disseminate critical information. And they fended off attacks on science and their profession, quashing misinformation at every turn.

These efforts saved countless lives in addition to giving public health a long-overdue boost in recognition. Because of the pandemic, people are beginning to appreciate the breadth and functions of public health. It's been heartening to see the public develop a better understanding of epidemiology and surveillance and use terms like *contact tracing* in everyday conversations. But improving awareness of public health during emergencies isn't enough to achieve bold population health goals. The COVID-19 pandemic has underscored that communication is not simply nice to have in public health but essential to its mission. It's time for public health to embrace communication and its possibilities for transforming practice.

Communication affects every aspect of public health, for better or worse. Nearly all public health practitioners have encountered a situation where communication—or the lack of it—has affected their work, and it's critical for the field to get it right every time. For health departments and other public health agencies, this means making communication an integral part of the overall organizational strategy, intertwined with administration, community engagement, and direct services. Giving communication a bigger platform may not be a welcome recommendation to an already overwhelmed public health department, but this doesn't need to be a burden. Leading with communication instead of treating it as an afterthought will ultimately benefit institutions of public health, enabling them to carry out their work more effectively and efficiently.

Communication is a team effort, requiring all members of an organization to participate. Even public health agencies that are fortunate enough to have communication experts on staff can't rely solely on these employees to handle messaging or outreach. That doesn't mean a harm reduction specialist has to become an expert in marketing or public relations. Rather, people with various skill sets can identify opportunities to bring communication into their work. For example, a health promotion campaign will go further with a social media strategy, while a behavioral intervention is more likely to succeed when practitioners employ a range of culturally competent messaging.

Embedding communication within the fabric of an organization is about more than increasing funding or bolstering a department's reputation, although those are certainly positive outcomes. Most important is how health agencies leverage communication to foster connections and help communities thrive. Being able to communicate about public health leads to deeper relationships within and outside of organizations: When going around the table for introductions at a multidisciplinary meeting, explain how each representative's unique skill set benefits a partnership or joint project. When speaking with residents, point to the risks or benefits to population health. At town halls, help city council members understand how their constituents benefit from sustained funding for public health.

Nontraditional sectors and community partners increasingly are thinking about health at the population level and are realizing the consequences of a society without a solid public health infrastructure. They can be part of the solution if they understand what public health is, its relevance to their own lives, and what their place in the system looks like. Now more than ever, public health needs the support of these diverse partners. And building bridges starts with effective communication that uses proven strategies.

Getting to a place where public health is widely understood and valued won't be easy. It takes time and patience to communicate across sectors in a way that will foster long-term collaboration. Be vigilant in helping people see the connections between public health and what matters to them most, whether that's creating safer neighborhoods or developing economic opportunities at the local level.

Public health finds itself in a difficult position, needing to address fallout from the pandemic and at the same time ensure that the field is neither sidelined nor marginalized in years to come. This is a critical juncture, and how we communicate will affect our ability to improve the health of communities and the nation. While we work to overcome the worst health crisis of the past century, we must deal with the consequences of decades of under-resourcing and underinvestment, which have led to elimination of jobs across public health. Communication will not solve all these long-standing problems, but it will be vital in navigating such complex territory.

The work of public health will always be necessary, even as crises abate. And that means that leaders continuously need to make the case for public health. With inspiration from this book, you can more confidently and more effectively articulate the needs of your organization and the overarching public health system.

Take what you have learned about framing, storytelling, and messaging and put this knowledge into action. Even if you have to start small, applying the principles of communication to your work can effect change that reverberates throughout the field. Don't underestimate the power of a personal dispatch from the frontlines or a thought-provoking, data-driven presentation to community leaders.

We can't afford to let our work recede into the background. To meet the challenges ahead, practitioners will need to employ all the tools at their disposal, especially the ones that have been underutilized. Communication is a means of preserving, protecting, and promoting public health, so embrace it in all that you do.

References

Introduction

1. Centers for Disease Control and Prevention, *MMWR: Morbidity and Mortality Weekly Report* 48, no. 12 (1999), https://www.cdc.gov/mmwr/PDF/wk/mm4812.pdf.
2. Centers for Disease Control and Prevention, "Ten Great Public Health Achievements—United States, 1900–1999," *MMWR: Morbidity and Mortality Weekly Report* 48, no. 12 (1999): 241–243, www.cdc.gov/mmwr/preview/mmwrhtml/00056796.htm.
3. Lauren Weber, Laura Ungar, Michelle R. Smith, The Associated Press, Anna Maria Berry-Jester, Hannah Recht, et al., "Hollowed-Out Public Health System Faces More Cuts Amid Virus," *Kaiser Health News*, August 24, 2020, khn.org/news/us-public-health-system-underfunded-under-threat-faces-more-cuts-amid-covid-pandemic/.
4. Michelle R. Smith, The Associated Press, and Lauren Weber, "Public Health Officials Are Quitting or Getting Fired in Throes of Pandemic," *Kaiser Health News*, August 11, 2020, khn.org/news/public-health-officials-are-quitting-or-getting-fired-amid-pandemic/.
5. Michelle R. Smith, The Associated Press, Lauren Weber, and Hannah Recht, "Public Health Experts Worry about Boom-Bust Cycle of Support," *Kaiser Health News*, July 21, 2021, khn.org/news/article/public-health-experts-worry-about-boom-bust-cycle-of-support/.
6. Kansas Department of Health and Environment, *Public Health Connections, Bureau of Community Health Systems* 15, no. 9 (2015), https://www.kdheks.gov/olrh/PH_Connections/Connect09-15.pdf.

7. Brian C. Castrucci, Ruth J. Katz, and Nat Kendall-Taylor, "Misunderstood: How Public Health's Inability To Communicate Keeps Communities Unhealthy," *Health Affairs Blog*, October 8, 2020, https://www.healthaffairs.org/do/10.1377/forefront.20201006.514 216/full/.

8. de Beaumont Foundation and Association of State and Territorial Health Officials, *Public Health Workforce Interests and Needs Survey: 2017 Findings* (de Beaumont Foundation, 2019), https://debeaumont.org/wp-content/uploads/2019/04/PH-WINS-2017.pdf.

Chapter 2

1. Milton Rokeach, *The Nature of Human Values* (New York: Free Press, 1973).

2. Paul M. Sniderman and Sean M. Theriault, "The Structure of Political Argument and the Logic of Issue Framing," in *Studies in Public Opinion: Attitudes, Non-attitudes, Measurement Error, and Change*, eds. W. E. Saris and P. M. Sniderman (Princeton, NJ: Princeton University Press, 2004), 133–165.

3. Lynn Davey, "How to Talk About Children's Mental Health: A FrameWorks Message Memo," FraemWorks Institute (December 2010), https://www.frameworksinstitute.org/wp-content/uploads/2020/03/CMH_MM.pdf.

4. Adam F. Simon, Nathaniel Kendall-Taylor, and Eric Lindland, "Using Values to Build Public Understanding and Support for Environmental Health Work," FrameWorks Institute (May 2013), https://www.frameworksinstitute.org/wp-content/uploads/2020/03/EnvironmentalHealth_values_final.pdf.

Index

patterns in important
information, seeing, 89
PHRASES (Public Health
Reaching Across Sectors),
4–5, 53, 99, 100
resource library, 100
policy change, framing as
key to, 29
positive outlook, 66, 92
power pitch(es), 113–14
crafting your, 114–15
prevention, 73*f*, 74–75
problems
focusing on problems
doesn't lead people to
solutions, 35
opening your eyes to the
problem, 94
problem statement, 114
public documents, 120–22,
121*f*, 122*f*
public health, 24. *See also* health;
specific topics
connotations of the term,
3–4, 14
defining, 15
functions, 73–75
importance, 24 (*see also*
urgency)
is not top-of-mind, 15
nature of, 106
negatively stereotyped
as siloed and "book
smart," 16–17
perceptions of
gaps between insiders and
other leaders', 9–10, 12*f*
views of leaders and
professionals outside
public health, 11,
19, 20*f*

transformation of, to meet
21st-century needs, 64, 92
public health impact
formula, 73–75
public health leaders. *See* l
eaders
public health narratives
to break down silos, 79–86
narrative development, 81
narrative structure, 75–77, 81
Public Health Reaching Across
Sectors. *See* PHRASES
Public Health Story Map, 93*f*
how to craft strategic
stories, 92–95
storytelling insights for sector-
specific audiences, 91–92

questions, answers to tough, 100

repeating what we want people
to forget doesn't shift
thinking, 33–34
research, relying on, 107
resources, 99–100

sectors, 64. *See also* cross-sector
collaborations; PHRASES;
social determinants
of health
data expertise helping
them find innovative
solutions, 66
demonstrating familiarity with
the sectors you wish to
engage, 63
role played by different, 84
sector-specific audiences,
storytelling insights
for, 91–92
simplicity. *See* complexity